CAMPYLOBACTERIOSIS

Anthrax

Campylobacteriosis

Cholera

HIV/AIDS

Influenza

Lyme Disease

Malaria

Mononucleosis

Polio

Smallpox

Syphilis

Toxic Shock Syndrome

Tuberculosis

Typhoid Fever

DEADLY DISEASES AND EPIDEMICS

CAMPYLOBACTERIOSIS

Bibiana Law

CONSULTING EDITOR
The Late **I. Edward Alcamo**
Distinguished Teaching Professor of Microbiology,
SUNY Farmingdale

FOREWORD BY
David Heymann
World Health Organization

CHELSEA HOUSE
P U B L I S H E R S
A Haights Cross Communications Company
Philadelphia

Dedication

We dedicate the books in the DEADLY DISEASES AND EPIDEMICS series to Ed Alcamo, whose wit, charm, intelligence, and commitment to biology education were second to none.

CHELSEA HOUSE PUBLISHERS

VP, NEW PRODUCT DEVELOPMENT Sally Cheney
DIRECTOR OF PRODUCTION Kim Shinners
CREATIVE MANAGER Takeshi Takahashi
MANUFACTURING MANAGER Diann Grasse

Staff for Campylobacteriosis

ASSOCIATE EDITOR Beth Reger
PRODUCTION EDITOR Megan Emery
PHOTO EDITOR Sarah Bloom
SERIES DESIGNER Terry Mallon
COVER DESIGNER Keith Trego
LAYOUT 21st Century Publishing and Communications, Inc.

©2004 by Chelsea House Publishers,
a subsidiary of Haights Cross Communications.

A Haights Cross Communications Company

http://www.chelseahouse.com

First Printing

1 3 5 7 9 8 6 4 2

Library of Congress Cataloging-in-Publication Data

Law, Bibiana, 1973–
    Campylobacteriosis/Bibiana Law.
       p. cm.—(Deadly diseases and epidemics)
    ISBN 0-7910-7899-X
    1. Campylobacter infections. I. Title. II. Series.
QR201.C25L39 2004
616.9'2—dc22

                                                         2004003296

Table of Contents

Foreword

In the 1960s, many of the infectious diseases that had terrorized generations were tamed. After a century of advances, the leading killers of Americans both young and old were being prevented with new vaccines or cured with new medicines. The risk of death from pneumonia, tuberculosis (TB), meningitis, influenza, whooping cough, and diphtheria declined dramatically. New vaccines lifted the fear that summer would bring polio, and a global campaign was on the verge of eradicating smallpox worldwide. New pesticides like DDT cleared mosquitoes from homes and fields, thus reducing the incidence of malaria, which was present in the southern United States and which remains a leading killer of children worldwide. New technologies produced safe drinking water and removed the risk of cholera and other water-borne diseases. Science seemed unstoppable. Disease seemed destined to all but disappear.

But the euphoria of the 1960s has evaporated.

The microbes fought back. Those causing diseases like TB and malaria evolved resistance to cheap and effective drugs. The mosquito developed the ability to defuse pesticides. New diseases emerged, including AIDS, Legionnaires, and Lyme disease. And diseases which had not been seen in decades re-emerged, as the hantavirus did in the Navajo Nation in 1993. Technology itself actually created new health risks. The global transportation network, for example, meant that diseases like West Nile virus could spread beyond isolated regions and quickly become global threats. Even modern public health protections sometimes failed, as they did in 1993 in Milwaukee, Wisconsin, resulting in 400,000 cases of the digestive system illness cryptosporidiosis. And, more recently, the threat from smallpox, a disease believed to be completely eradicated, has returned along with other potential bioterrorism weapons such as anthrax.

The lesson is that the fight against infectious diseases will never end.

In our constant struggle against disease, we as individuals have a weapon that does not require vaccines or drugs, and that is the warehouse of knowledge. We learn from the history of science that "modern" beliefs can be wrong. In this series of books, for example, you will learn that diseases like syphilis were once thought to be caused by eating potatoes. The invention of the microscope set science on the right path. There are more positive lessons from history. For example, smallpox was eliminated by vaccinating everyone who had come in contact with an infected person. This "ring" approach to smallpox control is still the preferred method for confronting an outbreak, should the disease be intentionally reintroduced.

At the same time, we are constantly adding new drugs, new vaccines, and new information to the warehouse. Recently, the entire human genome was decoded. So too was the genome of the parasite that causes malaria. Perhaps by looking at the microbe and the victim through the lens of genetics we will be able to discover new ways to fight malaria, which remains the leading killer of children in many countries.

Because of advances in our understanding of such diseases as AIDS, entire new classes of anti-retroviral drugs have been developed. But resistance to all these drugs has already been detected, so we know that AIDS drug development must continue.

Education, experimentation, and the discoveries that grow out of them are the best tools to protect health. Opening this book may put you on the path of discovery. I hope so, because new vaccines, new antibiotics, new technologies, and, most importantly, new scientists are needed now more than ever if we are to remain on the winning side of this struggle against microbes.

David Heymann
Executive Director
Communicable Diseases Section
World Health Organization
Geneva, Switzerland

1

David, Then Emma: What Is Happening to Me?

David woke up abruptly at 1:00 A.M. with severe stomach pain. He realized that if he did not rush to the bathroom, he would soon have an accident. Disoriented, he hurried to the bathroom. He had abdominal cramps and watery diarrhea. He felt warmer than normal and his muscles ached, but he was still sleepy so he went back to bed and was able to sleep until his alarm went off at 6:30 A.M.

David awoke with a mild headache but it was not too bad, and he decided to go to work. He prepared himself for work but ate only a small bowl of cereal due to some slight nausea. By noon, his headache was worse and he had to make another trip to the bathroom for more watery stools. David hated going to the doctor but decided to visit the pharmacy after work, especially since his headache was getting worse and his abdominal cramps were returning.

Upon arriving home, he took two tablets of Kaopectate® and two tablets of Tylenol® to help alleviate his **symptoms**. He had no appetite for dinner and still felt nauseated, but did manage to eat a little.

Nearing the end of a day dominated by nausea and diarrhea, David wondered if something he ate was causing all these problems. However, both he and his wife, Emma, ate the same foods the day before, except for lunch, and Emma was feeling fine. He shared lunch with some coworkers, who were also all healthy.

David had another bout of diarrhea that night. He took more Kaopectate and felt fatigued. He climbed back into bed and was able to fall asleep, but woke up again at 3:30 A.M. to run to the bathroom. He also had a fever of 100°F.

When David woke up the next morning, his head was spinning. He decided to work from home. However, after only a couple of hours of work, he was exhausted. He climbed back into bed but 45 minutes later had to get up due to another bout of diarrhea. His stools were loose and sticky and his abdominal cramps were getting worse. He vomited. Finally, he decided to see the doctor.

At the doctor's office, he explained his symptoms of abdominal cramps, diarrhea, nausea, fever, and now, vomiting. The doctor wrote up an order for a **stool sample**. The doctor explained to David that he probably had food poisoning, but that it is important to have the proper **diagnosis**, verified with laboratory samples. To be able to give an effective prescription, the doctor needed to know which pathogen was causing David's illness.

This is important because some **pathogens** have become resistant to certain **antibiotics**. Additionally, some **viruses** can cause **foodborne illness** with symptoms similar to bacterial **infections**, but viruses cannot be treated with antibiotics. With viruses, the disease must run its course. The doctor told David to monitor his fever, keep taking Tylenol, drink plenty of fluids, and come back first thing Friday for the diagnosis.

David brought the stool sample containers home and took a sample. Then he went to bed, absolutely exhausted. By Friday morning, David had not improved. He had seven or eight episodes of diarrhea the day before and his abdominal cramps got worse. Emma also had diarrhea. Her first bout was on Thursday afternoon.

David and Emma were both glad to see the doctor, who told them they have **campylobacteriosis**, an illness caused by the bacterium *Campylobacter* (pronounced "kamp-e-lo-back-ter"). *Campylobacter*, a bacterium most commonly found on raw

A WORD ON NOMENCLATURE

Nomenclature is a system of naming organisms based on concise and accurate descriptions. It allows scientists around the world to recognize and agree upon a standard name for a specific organism. Carolus Linnaeus, in the mid-18th century, developed a system called binomial nomenclature, which means that two words are used to describe an organism. Both words are derived from Latin. Every recognized species on Earth has a Latin binomial name. Latin was the language common to the educated people of the 1800s and, hence, it was used for nomenclature.

The binomial name for the bacterium that most commonly causes campylobacteriosis is *Campylobacter jejuni* (pronounced "kamp-e-lo-back-ter j-june-eye"). The first word, *Campylobacter*, capitalized and in italics, refers to the genus of the organism. The second word, also in italics, refers to the species of the organism. The genus refers to the larger category and includes the species in the same way that your last name includes all members of your family. Hence, *Campylobacter* refers to all *Campylobacter* species, such as *Campylobacter jejuni* and *Campylobacter coli* (abbreviated as *C. jejuni* and *C. coli*). Campylobacteriosis is the infectious disease caused by *Campylobacter* and does not need to be in italics.

In addition to species and genera, Linnaeus also developed other classificatory groups that are still used today. All organisms used to be divided into two basic kingdoms, Plantae and Animalia. Additional kingdoms such as Monera, Fungi, and Virus were added when it was clear that some organisms were not animals or plants. After the organisms were classified into kingdoms, they were further classified into phylum, class, order, family, genus, and species (Figure 1.1). Organisms were systematically grouped together based on related characteristics and compared in regard to anatomy, genetics, biochemistry, physiology, behavior, ecology, and geography.

For example, the Latin binomial name for humans is *Homo sapiens* (the genus is *Homo*). *Homo sapiens* are classified under the Kingdom Animalia, then Phylum Chordata, meaning animals with vertebra (spinal cord), then Class Mammalia, meaning mammals (warm-blooded animals that nourish their young with milk). Following is Order Primates (including humans, monkeys, apes, etc.), Family Hominidae, Genus *Homo*, and finally Species *Homo sapiens*, which is what we are.

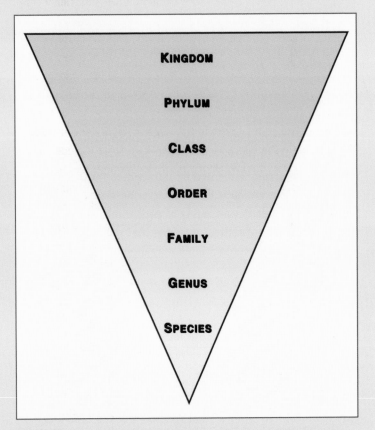

Figure 1.1 Organisms are divided into categories based on their characteristics. The broadest category is Kingdom, followed by the subcategories Phylum, Class, Order, Family, Genus, and Species.

poultry, unpasteurized milk, and untreated water, is a pathogen that causes **gastroenteritis**. David and Emma's abdominal cramps and diarrhea were caused by **inflammation** of the small intestine and large intestine due to the presence of the bacteria. The illness normally occurs 2 to 5 days after ingesting the contaminated food, which explains why Emma's diarrhea episodes did not begin until two days after David's. Emma had a longer **incubation period**. The illness generally lasts 5 to 10 days and, luckily for Emma, the antibiotics prescribed will shorten that period for her. Though the antibiotics will help David recover as well, he unfortunately has already suffered 3 to 4 days of diarrhea and abdominal cramps, not to mention the fever and vomiting.

FOODNET (CDC)

The FoodNet surveillance system was implemented to help resolve the severe underreporting of foodborne illnesses. FoodNet refers to the Foodborne Diseases Active Surveillance Network project implemented by the Centers for Disease Control and Prevention (CDC), which is the lead agency for protecting the health and safety of people in the United States. FoodNet is "active," meaning that public health officials frequently contact laboratory directors to find new cases of foodborne diseases to report electronically to CDC. Other surveillance systems are "passive," relying on clinical laboratories or patients to report foodborne diseases to state health departments, which in turn report to CDC, as with the case with David and Emma.

However, most patients, their physicians, and/or the laboratories fail to report foodborne illnesses. Sometimes, ill people do not seek medical attention. Other times, the physician fails to order a stool specimen or the laboratory fails to report the finding to CDC. FoodNet provides a solution for capturing unreported illnesses by actively watching for foodborne diseases and infections caused by bacteria such

The doctor explained that although fewer than 1 in 10 people inform the health department about such illness, reporting foodborne illnesses is important. He gave David and Emma the phone number to the County Environmental Services Department to report their foodborne illness. The doctor explained that the investigator would question them about what they ate up to 7 days before the onset of symptoms, how the food was prepared, and their activities, and would discuss with them the most probable source of the pathogen.

On Sunday, both David and Emma felt much better. It had been 48 hours since they started the antibiotics and though David still felt fatigued, his abdominal cramps were mild and the diarrhea episodes had tapered off. Emma felt fine since

as *Campylobacter, Salmonella, Shigella, Escherichia coli 0157,* and *Listeria monocytogenes*, and parasites such as *Cryptosporidium* and *Cyclospora.*

This project began in 1995 with five surveillance sites and has expanded to ten sites. So far, approximately 14% of the population in the United States is accounted for within these sites. The larger the population accounted for, the more accurate the statistics provided by FoodNet will be. FoodNet is a system that helps public health officials better understand the epidemiology (pattern and causes of disease) of foodborne diseases in the United States. For the public, FoodNet allows dissemination of information of disease trends. As well, the FoodNet website provides links to each state's Department of Health, which, in turn, provides health news and alerts along with where and how to report foodborne illnesses. Information acquired through FoodNet will allow foodborne disease trends to be monitored, which helps lead to new interventions and prevention strategies. For more information, go to: *http://www.cdc.gov/foodnet/default.htm.*

her illness was treated early. David was able to go to work on Monday and was relieved to have absolutely no diarrhea.

THE INFAMOUS *CAMPYLOBACTER*

Campylobacter is one of the leading causes of sporadic bacterial diarrheal illness in the United States (Figure 1.2). It is estimated to cause approximately 2.4 million cases per year, which is more than *Shigella* and *Salmonella* bacteria combined. Anyone can contract campylobacteriosis, but children under 5 years of age and young adults aged 15 to 29 years are most often afflicted.

Emma and the County Environmental Services Department staff deduced that the source of her and David's illness was probably the chicken they prepared for their Sunday dinner the weekend before they got sick. Emma grilled the chicken while David prepared the salad. Though the chicken was probably cooked properly because Emma remembered that she had over-cooked it, the investigator asserted that **cross-contamination** was the problem. Cross-contamination occurs when bacteria spreads from something that is contaminated to something that is not; in this case, bacteria spread from the raw chicken to the salad.

Only one drop of raw chicken juice is required to cause illness. Unlike some pathogens, *Campylobacter* requires an extremely small **infective dose**. Only 500 bacteria are required for some people to become ill. A **colony** the size of a pinprick contains at least one million bacteria.

In David and Emma's case, cross-contamination could easily have occurred if the sink was not properly **sanitized** after Emma took the chicken breasts out of their packages in the sink. Emma could also have splattered some of the chicken juices on the counter when she placed the chicken breasts on a plate before bringing them to the grill. David washed the lettuce and red peppers in the sink and cut and chopped them on a chopping board on the counter beside the sink, so there were plenty of opportunities for cross-contamination if proper sanitizing measures were not taken before making the salad.

Estimated illnesses, hospitalizations, and deaths caused by known foodborne pathogens, United States

Disease or agent	Illnesses			Hospitalizations			Deaths		
	Total	Food-borne	% of total foodborne	Total	Food-borne	% of total foodborne	Total	Food-borne	% of total foodborne
Bacterial									
Bacillus cereus	27,360	27,360	0.2	8	8	0.0	0	0	0.0
Botulism, foodborne	58	58	0.0	46	46	0.1	4	4	0.2
Brucella spp.	1,554	777	0.0	122	61	0.1	11	6	0.3
Campylobacter spp.	2,453,926	1,963,141	14.2	13,174	10,539	17.3	124	99	5.5
Clostridium perfringens	248,520	248,520	1.8	41	41	0.1	7	7	0.4
Escherichia coli O157:H7	73,480	62,458	0.5	2,168	1,843	3.0	61	52	2.9
E. coli, non-O157 STEC	36,740	31,229	0.2	1,084	921	1.5	30	26	1.4
E. coli, enterotoxigenic	79,420	55,594	0.4	21	15	0.0	0	0	0.0
E. coli, other diarrheogenic	79,420	23,826	0.2	21	6	0.0	0	0	0.0
Listeria monocytogenes	2,518	2,493	0.0	2,322	2,298	3.8	504	499	27.6
Salmonella typhi	824	659	0.0	618	494	0.8	3	3	0.1
Salmonella, nontyphoidal	1,412,498	1,341,873	9.7	16,430	15,608	25.6	582	553	30.6
Shigella spp.	448,240	89,648	0.6	6,231	1,246	2.0	70	14	0.8
Staphylococcus food poisoning	185,060	185,060	1.3	1,753	1,753	2.9	2	2	0.1
Streptococcus, foodborne	50,920	50,920	0.4	358	358	0.6	0	0	0.0
Vibrio cholerae, toxigenic	54	49	0.0	18	17	0.0	0	0	0.0
V. vulnificus	94	47	0.0	86	43	0.1	37	18	1.0
Vibrio, other	7,880	5,122	0.0	99	65	0.1	20	13	0.7
Yersinia enterocolitica	96,368	86,731	0.6	1,228	1,105	1.8	3	2	0.1
Subtotal	5,204,934	4,175,565	30.2	45,826	36,466	59.9	1,458	1,297	71.7
Parasitic									
Cryptosporidium parvum	300,000	30,000	0.2	1,989	199	0.3	66	7	0.4
Cyclospora cayetanensis	16,264	14,638	0.1	17	15	0.0	0	0	0.0
Giardia lamblia	2,000,000	200,000	1.4	5,000	500	0.8	10	1	0.1
Toxoplasma gondii	225,000	112,500	0.8	5,000	2,500	4.1	750	375	20.7
Trichinella spiralis	52	52	0.0	4	4	0.0	0	0	0.0
Subtotal	2,541,316	357,190	2.6	12,010	3,219	5.3	827	383	21.2
Viral									
Norwalk-like viruses	23,000,000	9,200,000	66.6	50,000	20,000	32.9	310	124	6.9
Rotavirus	3,900,000	39,000	0.3	50,000	500	0.8	30	0	0.0
Astrovirus	3,900,000	39,000	0.3	12,500	125	0.2	10	0	0.0
Hepatitis A	83,391	4,170	0.0	10,841	90	0.9	83	4	0.2
Subtotal	30,833,391	9,282,170	67.2	123,341	21,167	34.8	433	129	7.1
Grand Total	38,629,641	13,814,924	100.0	181,177	60,854	100.0	2,718	1,809	100.0

Figure 1.2 Many microorganisms, including bacteria, parasites, and viruses, cause foodborne illnesses. These organisms, and the number of illnesses they cause, are listed in this chart.

In summary, *Campylobacter* causes the highest incidence of bacterial illnesses. The majority of causes are attributed to foodborne illnesses, such as in David and Emma's case. Presently, handling and consumption of raw or improperly cooked poultry and cross-contamination are the most probable causes. However, there are other causative agents of *Campylobacter* and research is ongoing to determine other sources of campylobacteriosis. Foodborne illnesses can also be brought on by other causative agents, such as viruses, fungi, and parasites, which will be discussed in the next chapter.

2

Causative Agents of Infectious Diseases

Infectious diseases are caused by the infection of a host, such as humans, by infectious agents. Although *Campylobacter* is a **bacterium**, other infectious agents such as viruses, **fungi**, and **parasites** can also cause infectious diseases. **Disease** refers to the existence of **pathology** such as clinical symptoms or complications.

When the infectious agents invade the body and multiply, they cause harm to our bodies, which can be seen as symptoms (a change in condition as perceived by the patient) such as diarrhea, vomiting, or abdominal pain. These are called **clinical symptoms** because they are used to form a **clinical diagnosis**, which is made on the basis of knowledge obtained by medical history and physical examination, without confirmation by laboratory tests. The person presenting these symptoms is considered to have an infectious disease. To give a **definitive diagnosis**, a physician would require laboratory testing or X-rays to confirm the clinical diagnosis.

It is possible and common for people to be infected by an organism but be **asymptomatic** (presenting no symptoms of the disease). For example, people who are infected with parasitic worms, worms that live inside the body, often present no symptoms. This occurs with bacteria as well, including with *Campylobacter*, as certain individuals who come in contact with *Campylobacter* will shed the bacteria in their feces, indicating ingestion of the bacteria, but present no symptoms.

This severity of disease caused by an infectious agent is often described by **virulence**, which refers to the degree of abnormality caused by the infectious agent in a particular host, or the ability of the infectious agent to overcome the host's innate defenses or resistance to disease. The more virulent an infectious agent, the worse the clinical symptoms and complications will be.

Virulence not only depends on the innate characteristics of the infectious agent, but also on the host. Some infectious agents are **avirulent** in healthy people, but do cause disease, health complications, and even death in susceptible populations, such as infants, the elderly, or immunocompromised individuals such as those with acquired immunodeficiency syndrome (AIDS). For campylobacteriosis, for example, certain individuals, due to genetics, are predisposed to developing complications, such as reactive arthritis, which will be discussed in Chapter 4.

COMMON CAUSES OF INFECTIOUS DISEASES

This chapter provides descriptions of the microorganisms that cause infectious diseases, including bacteria, viruses, fungi, and parasites.

Bacteria

Although many bacteria are beneficial to us, they remain a major cause of disease. All bacteria belong to the prokaryotic kingdom Monera. Unlike more complex cells, bacteria do not have a membrane-bound **nucleus** or any intracellular organelles. Unlike fungi, plants, animals, or protozoa (which are **eukaryotic** and, therefore, larger and more complex), bacteria are much simpler (Figure 2.1).

Bacteria are unicellular and may be spherical, rod-like, or curved in their shape. Bacteria are the smallest living creatures, ranging in size from 0.1 micrometer (or micron) to 10 microns (a strand of human hair is 75 to 100 microns in diameter). The average bacterium is approximately 2 to 5 microns, whereas eukaryotic cells range from 2 to 100 microns. (100 microns equal one-tenth of 1 millimeter.)

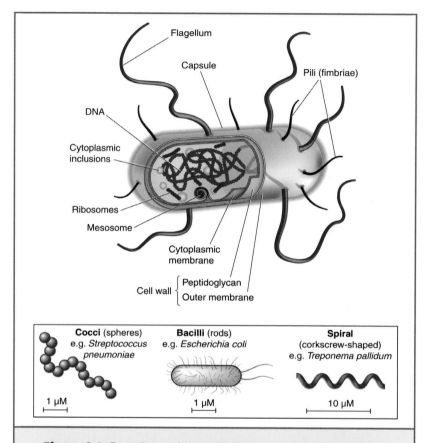

Figure 2.1 Bacteria are simple organisms in the Kingdom Monera. They do not have organelles or a membrane-bound nucleus. Some bacteria, such as *Campylobacter*, have flagella—little whip-like tails that help them move. Bacteria can also exist in three different shapes—cocci, bacilli, and spiral-shaped. Some of the common characteristics of bacteria are illustrated here.

Since bacteria are unicellular, they do not organize further into tissues but rather function independently. In contrast, human mucus-secreting cells and acid-secreting cells are organized into tissues such as the epithelial tissue lining the stomach. Tissues such as epithelial tissues, nervous tissues, and smooth muscle tissues are further organized into organs such as the stomach and the small and large intestines, which are then organized into systems such as the digestive tract. All the different systems such as the circulatory system, nervous system, digestive system, respiratory system, and so on work together to keep our bodies functioning properly.

SUSCEPTIBLE POPULATIONS

In the human population, there are subpopulations that are more vulnerable to disease than others. These are called **susceptible populations** and include infants, children, pregnant women, the elderly, and **immunocompromised** or **immunodeficient** individuals (people whose immune systems have been impaired or weakened, resulting in increased susceptibility to infections).

Infants are innately vulnerable because their immune systems are not fully developed. **Antibodies**, which are the body's fighters against foreign invaders, are not fully functional until approximately two and a half years of age. Maternal immune factors are transferred to the fetus via the **placenta** and to infants via breast milk to compensate for this delay in the immune system development. Thus, infants who are not breastfed are at higher risk for gastrointestinal and respiratory infections. Children are at higher risk due to increased exposure to infectious agents in dirt, playgrounds, and pets. Inadequate hygiene and improper sanitation contribute to the spread of infectious illness as well.

Pregnant women are considered to be at a higher risk due to the danger of passing the infection on to the fetus via the placenta and causing developmental deficiencies or death. The fetus develops at an extremely rapid rate in the uterus. In the first month, the fetal brain grows at a rate of 100,000 new brain cells per minute.[1] Any infection of the placenta can cause **placental insufficiency**, where inadequate transfer of oxygen, nutrients, and wastes can occur, thus causing

congenital malformations and death. Infection can also cause premature rupture of the membranes surrounding the fetus. Precautions need to be taken during pregnancy because certain infections that cause mild symptoms to the mother, such as the flu, can be detrimental or possibly even fatal to the fetus.

The elderly are considered a susceptible population because many elderly people are more prone to diseases such as cardiovascular disease or diabetes. Many are taking medications that cause **side effects**. It is much harder for the body to fight off infectious disease when it is continuously trying to repair itself from damage such as clogged arteries or weakened bones. The elderly also tend not to eat adequately and many do not get enough exercise, especially those in nursing homes. As a result, many elderly people do not have robust immune systems.

The immunocompromised subpopulation includes people whose immune systems are impaired or weakened by diseases such as AIDS or cancer. The immune system can also be impaired by medication or drugs, such as immunosuppressants that are given to transplant patients to suppress rejection of new organs. Some people are born with immunodeficiencies where their bodies are incapable of producing certain antibodies for protection. Others weaken their own immune system by partaking in habits such as drinking heavily, smoking, or eating poorly. For example, people who smoke are at higher risk for respiratory infections and lung cancer than those who do not smoke.

Bacteria, on the other hand are unicellular, and carry out all of their activities within one cell.

A bacterium's genetic material is also simple. It is organized into a single circular **chromosome** containing **deoxyribonucleic acid (DNA).** DNA contains all the genes that encode the bacterium's traits. This simplicity of design allows the genetic

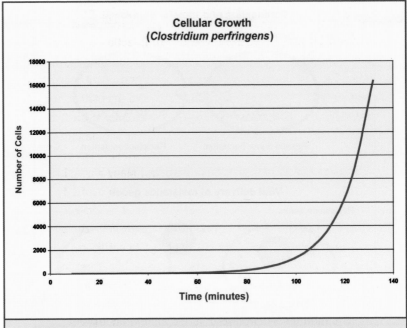

Figure 2.2 Bacteria reproduce at an exponential rate, as can be seen on this graph. Two cells of *Clostridium perfringes* will multiply to 16,000 cells in just over two hours.

material to be easily reproduced and also easily altered (mutated).

Favorable conditions such as warmth and availability of food will cause the cells to make a copy of their DNA and to grow larger until they are about double in size, at which point they divide into two identical cells with exact copies of the DNA. This is called **cell division**. The fastest-reproducing bacterium, *Clostridium perfringens*, doubles its numbers in approximately 8.8 minutes! Imagine how many *Clostridium perfringens* organisms there would be in 24 hours given favorable conditions (Figure 2.2).

Bacteria can alter their genetic material by three methods (Figure 2.3). Each method involves the transfer of small or large blocks of DNA, which allow the bacteria to acquire new traits that are beneficial to their survival (such as antibiotic

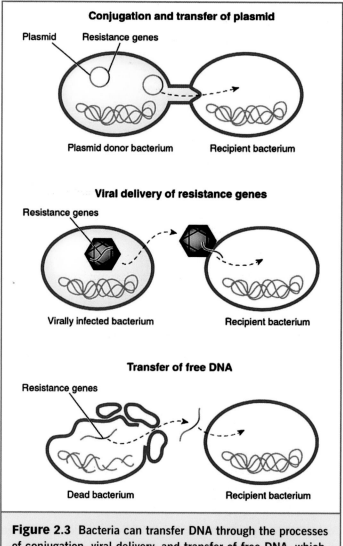

Conjugation and transfer of plasmid

Plasmid   Resistance genes

Plasmid donor bacterium   Recipient bacterium

Viral delivery of resistance genes

Resistance genes

Virally infected bacterium   Recipient bacterium

Transfer of free DNA

Resistance genes

Dead bacterium   Recipient bacterium

Figure 2.3 Bacteria can transfer DNA through the processes of conjugation, viral delivery, and transfer of free DNA, which lead to genetic variability that can aid in their survival. All three methods are illustrated here.

resistance, the ability to degrade new food sources, or the ability to avoid host defenses). *Campylobacter* is resistant to many antibiotics and has acquired these traits that allow it to survive via altering its own genetic material. The three methods are as follows:

- The first method of DNA transfer is called **conjugation**, which involves direct cell-to-cell contact. The donor cell transfers the DNA to the recipient cell via a **sex pilus**, which connects the two cells.

- The second method involves attaining new traits via a **bacteriophage** (a virus that attacks bacteria), which transfers DNA between bacteria in a process called **transduction**.

- The third method allows uptake of DNA from dead cells in the environment, a process called **transformation**.

The simplicity of bacteria's genetic material, the fact that bacteria are unicellular, and that they are small and can reproduce quickly allow them to thrive in many different types of environments. Although they are simpler in design than eukaryotes, they are exceedingly adaptable and can be found anywhere. They exist in the depths of the ocean, in the air and high in the atmosphere, in our soils, on our counters, on and inside our bodies—just about everywhere you can think of. A tablespoon of rich soil in a flowerpot can have billions of bacterial cells. Bacteria are diverse in their nutritional requirements; some can even use nonconventional items such as petroleum, paint, and rubber as food sources. They exist in astounding numbers and are ready to infect a host whenever the opportunity arises. *Campylobacter* is unique in that even though it is the number one cause of foodborne illness, we are still discovering new sources of infection. Campylobacteriosis is mainly associated with poultry products but research is indicating that pets and cattle (beef) may be sources as well. Though the versatility of *Campylobacter* allows it to thrive as an infectious agent, this trait of bacteria as a whole also allows other bacteria to be beneficial, such as the bacteria we use to make yogurt or those that maintain balance in the earth's environment.

Viruses

Viruses are unique organisms. They can multiply or replicate only inside the living cells of other animals, plants, or bacteria. They belong in their own kingdom and cannot truly be classified as a living entity because they remain dormant until they are in an appropriate host cell, unlike bacteria, which are able to live on their own outside the host. No free-living forms of viruses have been found.

Viruses are not composed of cells, which are considered to be the smallest structural unit of living matter that is able to function independently. Viruses have the genetic material but they absolutely need to borrow another cell's machinery in order to replicate (this concept is analogous to having an essay on a floppy disk but no computer to view it or a printer to print a copy). Viruses consist of genetic material and a protein shell called a **capsid** (Figure 2.4). Some viruses have an additional outer envelope, rod, and/or tail. Once inside a host, they utilize the host cell's machinery to create new viruses. Eventually, so many new viruses accumulate in the host cell that the cell ruptures. Then, the virus moves to another cell and repeats the process, causing more cell death and spreading infectious disease.

Viruses are extremely small and have a very simple composition. They range in size from 0.02 to 0.4 microns, smaller than bacteria. Viruses vary in their degree of virulence and ability to cause illnesses such as the common cold, caused by the influenza virus, to fatal diseases such as AIDS, caused by HIV (human immunodeficiency virus).

Fungi

Fungi include all organisms in the Kingdom Fungi, such as yeasts, molds, mushrooms, and mildews. Fungi are eukaryotic, multicellular organisms. The term *eukaryotic* refers to any cell or organism with cells that have a clearly defined nucleus. This nucleus is composed of a nuclear membrane that encloses the chromosomes. The chromosomes contain the genetic

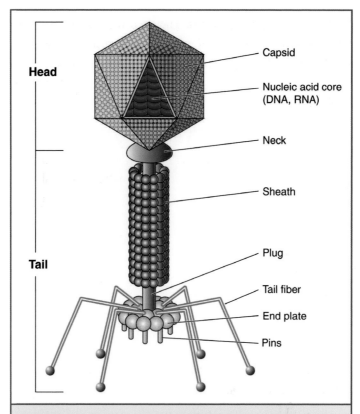

Figure 2.4 Viruses are composed of genetic material and a protein coat. One example of a virus, a bacteriophage, is illustrated here. Note that the genetic material (nucleic acid core) is coated with a protein capsid. Viruses do not have the means to reproduce on their own.

material DNA. Also, the **cytoplasm,** which is the material that fills the rest of the cell, contains various membrane-bound structures such as **mitochondria** that create and convert energy, a **Golgi apparatus** that modifies and transports proteins, and **lysosomes** that digest polysaccharides or old cell parts. Bacteria such as *Campylobacter* are prokaryotes, hence simpler in design, and have their DNA floating in their cytoplasm rather than being enclosed in a membrane.

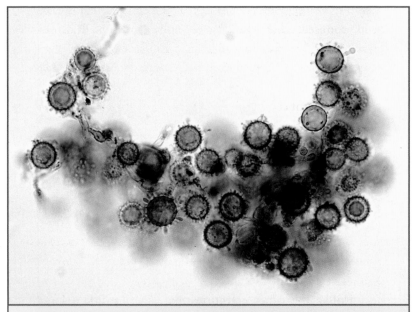

Figure 2.5 Fungi are eukaryotic, multicelluar, spore-forming organisms. A photomicrograph of the fungus *Histoplasma capsulatum* is shown here.

Although fungi are similar to plants, they are not considered plants because they do not contain the chlorophyll needed for **photosynthesis**, the process by which light energy is converted to chemical energy, which is an essential process for plants. Fungi also lack plant structures such as leaves, roots, or stems.

Out of the approximately 70,000 recognized species of fungi, only about 300 are known to cause human infections. In healthy people, fungi rarely cause disease, but in immunocompromised people, fungal infection can be fatal. An example of an infectious disease caused by fungi is histoplasmosis, caused by the fungus *Histoplasma capsulatum* (Figure 2.5). *H. capsulatum* is found worldwide, including in the United States, mainly in the eastern and central areas where soil is contaminated with bird or bat droppings. If the contaminated soil is disturbed, the **spores** become airborne. Inhaling the spores causes lung infections.

For more vulnerable people such as the elderly or immuno-compromised, other organs can become infected and death can result. Note, however, that all living organisms have their place and there are many beneficial fungi, with the most notable one being the *Penicillium* mold, from which penicillin, an antibiotic agent commonly used to treat bacterial infections in humans, is derived.

Parasites

Parasites are organisms that live on or within the host and gain sustenance from it. Three major groups of parasites cause human infections: the parasitic **protozoa**, the parasitic **helminthes** or worms, and certain **arthropods** (insects) that either directly cause disease or proceed as **vectors** (organisms that carry a pathogen that is the specific cause of disease).

Unlike the other categories, parasites include a large number of vastly different organisms. Viruses, fungi, and bacteria are considered parasites as well when they are living on or within the host while gaining sustenance. Generally, when referring to a parasitic infection, we mean one of these three groups: protozoa, worms, and insects (Figures 2.6). Other infections from viruses, fungi, and bacteria are referred to as viral infections, fungal infections, and bacterial infections, respectively.

Protozoa

Protozoa are unicellular eukaryotes. Their sizes range from microscopic to several millimeters in length. Protozoa include the **amoebas**, with their ability to form temporary cytoplasmic extensions called **pseudopodia** (commonly called false feet); flagellates, with their **flagella** (whip-like appendages); and **ciliates**, whose cell surface is covered with hundreds of hair-like structures called **cilia**. These protozoa differ significantly in their physiology and **life cycles**, and can be found in many soils and natural waters.

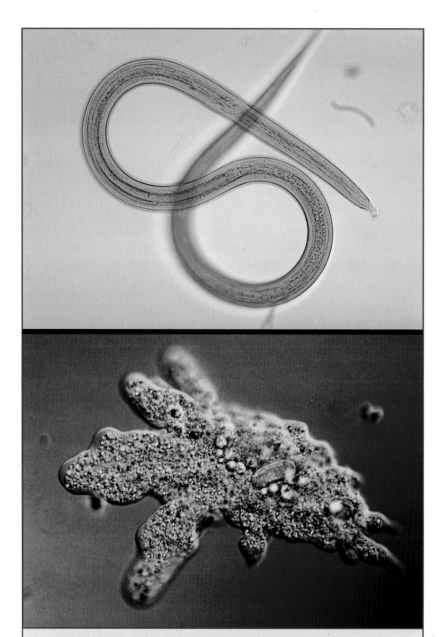

Figure 2.6 Parasitic worms (top) such as tapeworms and round-worms, and protozoa such as amoebas (bottom) can both cause human infections.

An example is the flagellate *Giardia intestinalis*, which causes an infectious disease known as giardiasis. Symptoms include severe diarrhea and malabsorption of nutrients, which can lead to debilitation with chronic giardiasis. Infection occurs when the **cysts** (similar to spores of bacteria) of *Giardia intestinalis* in contaminated water or food are ingested. The cysts revert back to the active form of *Giardia intestinalis* in the intestines (undergo the process of **excystment**). They then multiply and cause infection.

Worms

The parasitic helminthes, include the trematodes (flukes), cestodes (tapeworms), and nematodes (roundworms). "Helminth" is a general term for parasitic worms. Parasitic worms are quite large compared to bacteria. They range from 1 millimeter to over 15 meters (or 50 feet). They are multicellular eukaryotes, have well-developed organ systems, and most are active feeders. Depending on the type of worm, infection occurs due to ingestion of the eggs (**larvae**) or meat of the intermediate hosts that are involved in the life cycle of the worm, penetration of the skin by larvae, or exposure to bites of vectors (insects). Parasitic worms are found worldwide, especially in areas without adequate sanitation. Parasitic worms can easily live in the body for several years.

Insects

Parasites can have complex life cycles that involve vectors and **intermediate hosts**. A vector is an organism, typically an insect, which transmits the pathogen. A pathogen can then reside and multiply in an intermediate host, such as another insect. Therefore, an insect can serve as both an intermediate host and a vector for a pathogen.

An example of a disease caused by a vector is malaria, caused by a protozoan called plasmodia, which has a complex life cycle with various stages. Infected mosquitoes inject the sporozoites, a mature form of the protozoan that resides in the salivary glands of the mosquito, into the human host during feeding. These sporozoites invade the liver, mature further, and burst to release thousands of merozoites, which infect the red blood cells.

Insects can also be parasites by causing disease directly rather than being an intermediate host or vector. An example of causing direct disease is the head louse, *Pediculus humanus capitis*, an insect whose only hosts are humans. These head lice live on the scalp of humans and feed on the blood several times a day.

CAN YOUR CAT GIVE YOU AN INFECTION FROM A PROTOZOAN?

Cats are the main **reservoirs** of the protozoan *Toxoplasma gondii*. These protozoa live and multiply in the cat without harming the animal. Domesticated cats that kill and eat infected rodents, small animals, or birds are at higher risk for becoming infected with this protozoan, which can then be transmitted to humans.

Toxoplasma gondii causes a disease in humans called toxoplasmosis. This disease usually presents no symptoms in healthy people; if there are any symptoms, they are flu-like and include muscle aches and swollen lymph glands. Those whose immune systems are unable to fight the parasite can suffer from eye and brain damage due to the affinity of the parasite for these tissues.

Pregnant women need to take special precautions to prevent toxoplasmosis. Infants born to mothers who have become infected for the first time during or just before pregnancy are at the highest risk. Stillbirths can occur and, if the organism crosses the placenta and infects the fetus, the parasite can cause deafness and damage the retina of the eyes or brain (mental retardation) of the fetus. For those women planning to become

BENEFICIAL ASPECTS OF INFECTIOUS AGENTS

Although much emphasis has been placed on diseases caused by infectious agents, it is important to know that bacteria, viruses, fungi, and parasites also possess many beneficial traits.

Examples of beneficial bacteria include those found in the **flora** of our intestines. These bacteria protect us against the **colonization** of pathogenic bacteria. Other useful bacteria are those cultivated for use in wastewater treatment systems to decompose sewage, and those used to make yogurts and cheeses.

pregnant, blood tests can confirm if the mother has ever had toxoplasmosis. If the test is positive (indicating that the mother has had prior infection), there is no need to worry about passing the infection on to the baby because the mother will have already developed immunity. If the test is negative, precautions need to be taken to avoid infection since it is the first infection during the pregnancy that is dangerous.

Since cats become infected by eating other small animals, one can prevent infection by keeping the cat indoors. Other precautions include avoiding touching stray cats and kittens and changing the cat's litter every day. Since the parasite does not become infective for 1 to 5 days after it is released in the feces, cleaning the cat litter daily will prevent the parasite from becoming infectious in the home.

Cats rarely have symptoms, so it is not possible to know whether or not they have been infected. They normally pass *Toxoplasma* in their feces for only a few weeks and are fine to handle after those weeks pass. Since it is unknown when cats are infected, basic sanitation practices should always be followed, such as wearing gloves when dealing with soil or cleaning animal quarters.

Viruses, fungi, mold, and parasites can also be put to good use. Viruses that attack bacteria have been used in Europe for many years as alternatives to antibiotics. There are also beneficial fungi such as the mushrooms that many of us

THIRTY PERCENT OF THE WORLD'S POPULATION IS INFECTED BY THE NEMATODE *ASCARIS LUMBRIDOIDES*

Ascaris lumbridoides is the largest roundworm known to parasitize the small intestine of humans. Infection begins with ingestion of foods or soils contaminated with *Ascaris* eggs, typically raw fruits and vegetables grown in or near soil fertilized with sewage. Infected people who work with food can also contaminate a wide variety of foods if proper sanitation procedures are not followed.

After the eggs are swallowed, the larvae, which are the early form of the animal after hatching, invade the intestinal walls, enter the bloodstream, and travel to the lungs. They remain in the lungs and mature in 10 to 14 days, before ascending to the throat via the bronchial tree, to be swallowed once again. In the small intestine, they fully develop into adult worms to produce eggs that are passed with the feces to begin the cycle again. A female is capable of producing 200,000 eggs per day!

Symptoms are usually not seen when the worms are in their adult stage, although a high number of worms in the body may cause abdominal pain and intestinal obstruction. Migrating larvae can cause fever, coughing, shortness of breath, and pulmonary inflammation. Migration of adult worms can cause inflammation of the bile ducts and pancreas. Adult worms can reach up to 16 inches in length. Diagnosis is typically via microscopic examination of the stools for eggs, though adult worms are occasionally seen in the stools or found in the throat, mouth, or nose. Treatment is with drugs and, on occasion, surgery, if obstruction has occurred.

enjoy. Penicillin, a widely used antibiotic, is derived from the *Penicillium* mold. Even parasites contribute tremendously to maintaining the health of our soils. Our world cannot exist without these organisms.

SUMMARY

Although this book is about campylobacteriosis, an infectious disease caused by the bacteria *Campylobacter,* many different types of infectious agents, including viruses, fungi, and parasites, can cause diseases. The term *virulence* refers to the degree of the abnormality caused by the infectious agent in a particular host, or the ability of the infectious agent to overcome the host's innate defenses or resistance. It is important to remember as we go on to discuss campylobacteriosis that disease is not a one-way street, but rather a dynamic interplay between the host and the invading agent. The role of medicine is to give the benefit to the host. Although bacteria, viruses, fungi, and parasites can be infectious agents, they also possess beneficial traits and give us many of the things that we need and enjoy.

3
Campylobacteriosis: An Infectious Disease

Campylobacteriosis is the term referring to the infectious disease caused by bacteria of the genus *Campylobacter*. Veterinarians have long recognized that *Campylobacter* causes diarrhea and spontaneous abortions in cattle and sheep. For many decades, people erroneously believed that *Campylobacter* did not affect humans. However, since the 1980s, there has been an increasing awareness that more research needs to be conducted on *Campylobacter*. This is due to the findings of FoodNet indicating high numbers of human infections, estimated to be close to 2.4 million cases per year (which is equivalent to approximately 1% of the population of United States!) Additionally, *Campylobacter* has been found to be the most common infection preceding Guillain-Barré syndrome, the leading cause of acute neuromuscular paralysis.

Campylobacteriosis is considered a **zoonosis**, a disease that can be passed from animals to humans under natural conditions. Among animals, the most common form of transmission is via the **fecal-oral route**. The bacteria are shed in the feces of one animal and are then ingested by another. This does not necessarily mean that the recipient animal is directly eating the feces of the donor animal; more likely, the food or water ingested by the recipient animal has been contaminated by feces from an infected animal. In close quarters, feces can normally be found in cages, feed, and water bins. Retail chickens, normally caged close together and processed in high volumes, have contamination rates of over 50% and are suspected to be the primary source of campylobacteriosis in humans.

Although *Campylobacter* is the most frequently isolated bacterium in the laboratory for people with diarrhea (45%), other bacteria such as *Salmonella* (17%), *Shigella* (17%), and *E. coli 0157:H7* (5%) get much more media attention when they cause food poisoning.[2] This is because campylobacteriosis is a sporadic disease, not an outbreak type of disease.

CAMPYLOBACTER: THE ORGANISM

The *Campylobacter* species responsible for 90% of campylobacteriosis is *Campylobacter jejuni*. *C. jejuni* was once thought to be a rare and **opportunistic pathogen**, which attacked immunocompromised individuals but not those who had robust immune systems. *C. jejuni* is certainly a pathogen, but anyone can become infected, including healthy people of all ages. Even though anyone can be infected, the incidence is higher in children and young adults (ages 15 to 29). Certainly those who are immunocompromised are more at risk for serious complications. There is a slight predominance in males. Although the reason remains unknown, a study by M.S. Deming et al., (1987) indicated that one major factor among male students preparing food while residing in university housing in the United States was the consumption of poorly prepared and undercooked chicken.[3]

Campylos is a Latin term derived from the Greek word *kampylos*, which means "bent," and "bac" refers to *bacillus*, which means "rod-like." The organism is a spirally curved rod that has a flagellum at one or both ends of the cell (Figure 3.1). Flagella are extra-cellular hair-like appendages that the bacteria use to propel themselves by whip-like movements. This combination of being spiral-shaped and having flagella gives them their characteristic corkscrew-like motion. They are highly motile and will dart up, down, and across when viewed under a microscope. *Campylobacter* cells are very small, measuring 0.2 to 0.5 microns wide and 0.5 to 5 microns long. (Remember that 1 micron is 1/1,000 of a millimeter, or approximately

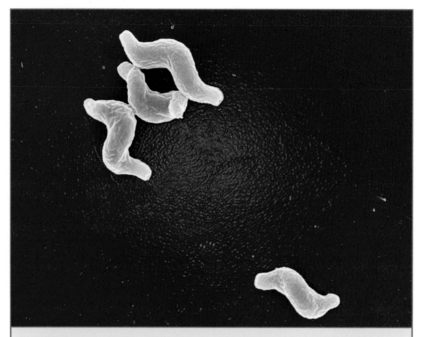

Figure 3.1 *Campylobacter jejuni*, shown here, is a Gram-negative spiral-shaped rod with flagella at one or both ends. They are less than 5 microns in length. Under stressful conditions, *Campylobacter jejuni* will form coccoid bodies.

1/25,000 of an inch. Imagine dividing 1 inch into 25,000 parts!) Unlike some microorganisms that form spores, which are the resistant form of the bacteria produced under adverse conditions, *Campylobacter* do not form spores as a mechanism to hibernate until favorable conditions appear again. *Campylobacter* cells do form **coccoid bodies** (become round), though, when under stress, but unlike spores, will eventually die if favorable conditions do not return.

CAMPYLOBACTER IN THE LABORATORY

Detection of *Campylobacter* has been difficult because the organisms are **microaerophilic**, which means that they require less oxygen and more carbon dioxide than **aerobic bacteria** for survival. For example, to grow *Campylobacter* in the laboratory, special **bacteriological incubators** are used to provide the necessary controlled environment. These insulated incubators regulate the air that is circulated inside to consist of 5–10% carbon dioxide and 5–10% oxygen, with the remainder as nitrogen. In addition, these incubators regulate the temperature at a constant at 42°C (107.6°F). The air we breathe and the conditions that aerobic bacteria prefer have a carbon dioxide content of 0.03%, an oxygen content of 21%, and a nitrogen content of approximately 79%.

Detection and isolation of *Campylobacter* from feces of infected patients requires special equipment and special **media** (the substance on which bacteria is grown in the laboratory). These techniques were not developed until the 1970s and continue to be improved today.

Campylobacter is a fragile organism that is sensitive to common environmental stresses such as drying, heating, **disinfectants** (such as chlorine bleach), and atmospheric air (21% oxygen). Also, since *Campylobacter* prefers to live at the warm temperature of 37–42°C (107.6°F), it will grow poorly (if at all) when refrigerated (normally 4°C or 39.2°F). However, *Campylobacter* will grow at room temperature (about 25°C or 77°F).

Once ingested, the human digestive system provides *Campylobacter* with the requirements it desires. Human intestines are basically **anaerobic** (lacking oxygen), with pockets where there is some oxygen (microaerophilic). The body also provides the warmth that *Campylobacter* requires in order to thrive.

INFECTION CLUSTERS

Most *Campylobacter* infections occur as sporadic single cases or family clusters. Outbreaks are quite rare but do occur, usually due to consumption of unpasteurized milk products or polluted water. The **incidence** of *Campylobacter* infections also

GRAM-NEGATIVE VS. GRAM-POSITIVE BACTERIA

The **Gram stain** is a technique used to classify bacteria based upon the characteristics of their cell membranes. In 1884, a Danish physician, Hans Christian Gram, discovered that a particular dye (crystal violet) would stain certain bacteria irreversibly but not others. Stains are used to help microbiologists identify and characterize bacteria because they allow cells to be visualized under a microscope. Since bacteria are so small, they are extremely difficult to see without some aid.

The Gram stain procedure consists of heat fixing a smear of bacterial cells on a slide over a flame, and then adding crystal violet. This stains the cells purplish blue. The slide is then washed with iodine, which forms an insoluble complex with the primary stain (crystal violet). Then, the slide is washed with an alcohol solution, which washes away the purplish blue stain in some bacteria but not in others. The slide is then stained with a counterstain, safranin. If the initial stain has been washed away, safranin turns the cells pinkish red.

Bacteria that stain purplish blue (and thus retain the initial stain) are called Gram-positive; bacteria that stain pinkish red are called Gram-negative (Figure 3.2). Gram-positive bacteria retain the blue color because they have much thicker cell walls consisting of up to 90% **peptidoglycan**, which is a polymer of sugar derivatives that help retain the blue stain. Gram-negative bacteria stain pinkish red because their cell wall consists of only approximately 10% peptidoglycan and is a thinner structure with distinct layers. Thus, alcohol can penetrate and wash out the crystal violet prior to staining with safranin. *Campylobacter* organisms are Gram-negative.

The Gram stain reflects the differences in the structural properties of bacteria and allows us to assign certain characteristics to certain bacteria. For example, the bacteria that naturally live on our skin, which is dry and slightly acidic, are mostly Gram-positive bacteria. This is logical because they need the thick cell wall so they do not dry out.

Gram-negative bacteria tend to be more pathogenic since the main component of their cell wall is **lipopolysaccharide (LPS)**, which is associated with endotoxic activity. In microbiology, the term *LPS* is used synonymously with **endotoxin**, a toxin that, when present in large numbers in our bloodstream, causes negative physiological reactions including fever, cardiopulmonary symptoms such as rapid breathing and shortness of breath (tachypnea), increased heart rate (tachycardia), and multiple organ failure, which eventually leads to death.

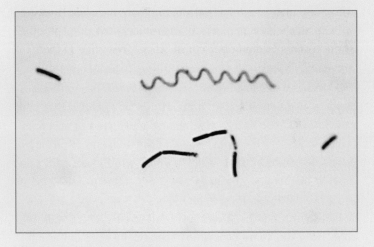

Figure 3.2 The Gram stain is a procedure that identifies bacteria based on the characteristics of their cell walls. Gram-positive organisms that retain the initial crystal violet stain and will appear bluish purple under the microscope. Bacteria that lose the initial stain but take up the counterstain, safranin, will appear pinkish red under the microscope and are designated Gram-negative. Both Gram-positive and Gram-negative bacteria are present in this photograph.

tends to be higher in the summer than in the winter. Some likely reasons include summer activities such as barbecuing foods and drinking untreated water from rivers or streams when hiking or camping.

Recall that campylobacteriosis is a zoonotic disease. No matter how pristine rivers or streams may look, animals such as birds eliminate feces in the water, thus contaminating it.

OUTBREAK OF *C. JEJUNI* INFECTIONS IN WISCONSIN, 2001

Unpasteurized milk is a common source of pathogens including *Campylobacter, Brucella, Escherichia coli, Salmonella, Listeria monocytogenes, Mycobacterium bovis,* and *Corynebacterium diphtheriae.* **Pasteurization** is the partial sterilization of a substance such as milk or juice to destroy pathogenic microorganisms without significantly altering the chemical composition of the products themselves. This is accomplished by exposing the product to high temperatures for specified amounts of time. The process was named after the famous French scientist Louis Pasteur, who demonstrated in the 1860s that heating beer and wine to 57°C (135°F) for a few minutes would prevent abnormal fermentation. In the United States, pasteurization of milk is accomplished by either heating to 63°C (145°F) and maintaining that temperature for 30 minutes, or heating to and holding at 72°C (162°F) for 15 seconds.

Pasteurization has long been used to ensure that milk is safe. However, some consumers specifically seek out unpasteurized milk because they believe that it tastes better, cures or prevents certain medical conditions, or offers enhanced nutrition. However, these claims have not been scientifically established.

This was the case recently in Wisconsin. In 2001, consumers could not purchase unpasteurized milk legally in Wisconsin. To circumvent regulations that prohibit the

SOURCES OF INFECTION

Campylobacter organisms live as **commensals** in the intestinal tracts of many birds and mammals, such as chickens, turkeys, ducks, cattle, and domesticated pets such as dogs (especially puppies) and cats. Living as commensals means that the *Campylobacter* organisms benefit from their host organism in terms of nutrients and shelter but do not substantially

sale of unpasteurized milk, certain farms established cow-leasing programs, where consumers could pay a fee for the milk produced by local cows. The milk from these cows was not pasteurized and was stored in a bulk holding tank. Consumers picked up this milk from the farm or had it delivered to their homes.

In avoiding pasteurization, 75 people acquired campylo-bacteriosis in northwestern Wisconsin in November and December of 2001. The symptoms reported were: diarrhea (in 93% of those afflicted), abdominal cramps (92%), fever (76%), nausea (40%), and bloody diarrhea (23%). Fortunately, none of the patients required hospitalization and none had complications. Of the 75 patients, 70 reported drinking unpasteurized milk, 4 reported not drinking unpasteurized milk but being mothers of ill children who drank unpasteur-ized milk, and 1 was categorized as having an unknown mode of infection.

Laboratory tests confirmed that strains of *C. jejuni* grown from unpasteurized milk samples from a particular organic Grade A dairy farm matched the strains from the feces of the patients who had campylobacteriosis. As a result, to ensure that unpasteurized milk will no longer be sold or distributed to consumers, cow-leasing programs are no longer legal in Wisconsin.[4]

affect the host. This is similar to how some strains of *E. coli* live in our intestines and use our nutrients but do not affect us in any noticeable manner. The bacteria use our nutrients but they do not use enough to cause any deficiencies.

In humans, *Campylobacter* organisms are not commensals; instead, they are pathogens and can cause infection and illness. However, some patients are asymptomatic, presenting no symptoms of the disease such as diarrhea or abdominal pain. They simply shed the bacteria in their feces and can contaminate food and water sources, just as the commensals in birds and mammals do. Since so many birds and mammals have a commensal relationship with *Campylobacter* organisms, the potential pathways of infection are many.

However, all of these sources of infection are minor when compared with food sources. Campylobacteriosis is essentially a foodborne disease with raw or undercooked meat being the principal vehicle of infection. Any type of raw meat can be contaminated with *Campylobacter*, but poultry is the most likely source, especially broiler chickens, since massive amounts are produced and consumed. The United States produces more than 8 billion broiler chickens a year. Retail chickens usually have contamination rates of over 50%. This does not mean that people should not consume chicken, as *Campylobacter* organisms are killed by heat during cooking. However, food handlers must be diligent. Cross-contamination from raw chickens to other foods during storage and preparation is a common source of infection.

INFECTIOUS DOSE
Campylobacter requires an extremely small infective dose. Only 500 bacteria are required for some people to become ill. (In comparison, some strains of *Salmonella* and *E. coli* have an infectious dose of more than 100,000 organisms.) However, although the infectious dose is low, person-to-person

transmission is low as well. This is one reason for the lack of outbreaks of campylobacteriosis.

At first, it seems logical that person-to-person transmission would be high since such a low infectious dose is required, but recall the sensitivity of *Campylobacter*. Outside of the intestinal tract, the lack of growth and poor survival of *Campylobacter* mean it has a low transmission rate. Once ingested, though, *Campylobacter* is quite capable of reproducing and causing damage. As with other food poisonings, the attack rate or degree of illness varies according to the ingested dose and the particular strain of bacteria. The higher the dose or more virulent the strain, the higher the chance for successful invasion and colonization of the small and large intestines, and ultimately, faster reproduction. Faster reproduction of these pathogenic organisms leads to more damage and more symptoms and complications. Of course, the ability of the host to fight back is an important factor in how sick he or she becomes.

4

Campylobacteriosis: Symptoms and Complications

SYMPTOMS

The foremost symptom in campylobacteriosis is **enteritis**, indicating inflammation of the intestines. *Campylobacter* enteritis manifests as an acute diarrheal disease with clinical symptoms, such as abdominal pain and fever. These clinical symptoms are similar to other bacterial gut infections such as salmonellosis from the bacteria *Salmonella enteritidis*, which is commonly found in eggs and poultry. A definitive diagnosis cannot be made from the clinical symptoms since the symptoms are so similar to other bacterial infections caused by food poisoning. To make an accurate diagnosis, the patient's feces must be examined in a laboratory. Recall David's case in Chapter 1 when he visited the doctor. He needed to wait two days for his diagnosis.

Most cases of campylobacteriosis begin with abrupt abdominal pains and diarrhea along with possible nausea, vomiting, muscle aches, fever, and headaches (Figure 4.1). Some patients do suffer from a non-specific flu-like **prodrome**, which is a premonitory symptom of disease consisting of one or more symptoms of fever, headache, dizziness, and muscle aches for 2 to 3 days prior to the abdominal pains and diarrhea. These cases tend to be more severe than those without the prodromal symptom.[5] Be aware, though, that there are a wide variety of symptoms, ranging from no symptoms (asymptomatic) to mild gastrointestinal

Characteristics of Campylobacteriosis

Organism	*Campylobacter jejuni*
Incubation Period	Typically 2–5 days
Signs and Symptoms	Diarrhea, cramps, fever, and vomiting; diarrhea may be bloody
Duration of Illness	2–10 days, typically 3–6 days
Associated Foods	Raw and undercooked poultry, unpasteurized milk, contaminated water
Laboratory Testing	Routine stool culture; *Campylobacter* requires special media and incubation at 37–42°C to grow.
Treatment	Supportive care. For severe cases, antibiotics such as erythromycin and quinolones may be indicated early in the diarrheal disease. Guillian-Barré syndrome can be a sequela.

Figure 4.1 The symptoms of campylobacteriosis include diarrhea, cramps, fever, and vomiting, and the illness can last anywhere from 2 to 10 days. Foods associated with the illness, tests to determine the diagnosis, and treatment options are shown in this table.

distress lasting a day or two, to a fulminating (explosive) enteritis or **colitis** that includes **hemorrhagic** (bleeding) inflammation and lesions. These more severe symptoms resemble **ulcerative colitis**, a painful chronic disease where the large intestine or colon is inflamed and covered with **ulcers** (holes that develop in the inflamed lining).

The diarrhea is usually profuse and watery. In approximately 15% of patients, the diarrhea turns bloody from the inflammation and lesions. Some patients have more than 10 **bowel movements** a day. A symptom that the enteritis is caused by

Campylobacter rather than other bacteria is intense and continuous abdominal pain, which can get so severe that the pain radiates to the right hip. This intense pain, mimicking **appendicitis**, is the most common reason for admissions into hospitals.[6]

After 3 to 4 days, the diarrhea lessens and the recovery stage begins. However, some patients have **relapses**, usually caused by eating too much. The digestive tract is not sufficiently healed and too much food can cause a recurrence of symptoms, especially abdominal pain. Weight loss of 10 pounds (4.5 kilograms) is not uncommon. Death is rare and is usually limited to those who are immunocompromised or the elderly.[7]

The usual incubation period, which is the time between exposure to the infectious agent and onset of the first symptom, is 2 to 5 days, but can take as long as 8 days. The duration of the illness is usually one week. In severe cases, the symptoms can persist for up to three weeks. Fluid and electrolyte replacement remain the cornerstone of treatment, just like for other diarrhea diseases. For mild symptoms, antibiotics are not required. Specific treatment with antibiotics is used for more severe or prolonged symptoms or for those who are immunocompromised. Untreated patients may shed the organisms in their feces for up to several months.

COMPLICATIONS

Complications are rare, but infections have been associated with bacteremia, most often in those whose immune systems are compromised. If untreated, these infections can lead to infections of any organ. Abortion and **perinatal infection**, and late-onset complications such as reactive arthritis (Reiter's syndrome) and Guillain-Barré syndrome (a rare neurological paralysis) occur only rarely.

Bacteremia

Bacteremia refers to the presence of bacteria in the bloodstream. Among patients who are healthy, bacteremia occurs as a transient event and the natural defenses of the body are able to kill the bacteria. Blood naturally contains agents to fight foreign invaders.

For the severely immunocompromised, however, **septicemia** can occur where the host loses the battle and the bacteria spread and cause infection of other organs, such as the heart or kidneys. Septicemia, also called blood poisoning, includes bacteria in the blood (bacteremia) and toxins from the bacteria circulating in the blood (toxemia). Septicemia, if not treated

ORAL REHYDRATION THERAPY

When suffering from diarrhea, it is important to replenish the fluids that are lost. This is especially critical for children and the elderly.

In many parts of the world, people suffer from chronic hunger. This chronic malnutrition eventually causes the individual's immune system to be compromised. Most children who die of malnutrition do not starve to death but die from being unable to fight infections that cause diarrhea from the food or water upon which they subsist. Improper sanitation and inadequate hygiene contribute to this infection-diarrhea cycle. To prevent death from severe diarrhea, world aid workers rely on **oral rehydration therapy**, which works by increasing the body's ability to absorb fluids. Oral rehydration therapy is estimated to save over a million lives each year.

Aid workers teach parents to make an oral fluid replace-ment from simple ingredients from home. A common recipe is 1 cup boiled or disinfected water, 2 teaspoons sugar, and a pinch of salt.[8] Sugar and salt help the water to be absorbed by the body (sport drinks work similarly). Of course, in some areas of developing countries, clean water may be difficult to obtain. In North America, though, this simple recipe can be used at home to help the body recover.

BACTEREMIC SHOCK

Bacteremic shock, a condition in which bacteria invade the bloodstream and cause the body to shut down, is most often caused by Gram-negative organisms due to the lipopolysaccharide (LPS) in their cell wall, which triggers a response from the immune system. The higher the amounts of LPS in the blood, the stronger the response will be. Shock usually occurs when the circulatory system is no longer able to supply enough blood to the surrounding tissues. Oxygen and nutrient requirements are not met, and wastes or toxins cannot be removed from the afflicted tissues. Consequently, the failure of organs such as the kidneys, brain, and lungs can lead to death.

The cause of bacteremic shock is widespread dilation of the blood vessels, which results in too little blood circulating throughout the system. Bacteremic shock occurs when the bacteria and/or their products reach such high levels in the bloodstream that an inflammatory response is triggered throughout the body, not just locally at the infected site.

Although the goal of an inflammatory response is to eliminate the foreign bodies, there is a cost to the body in which human tissue is destroyed and eliminated as well. At a localized site such as the small intestine, the area can heal if given time and rest. However, when the entire body is affected, this is a signal that the immune system is unable to take care of the infection. Immediate medical intervention is required.

Along with the dilation of the blood vessels, the inflammation in enteritis results in bloody diarrhea, which exacerbates the low blood volume due to loss of fluids and blood. The symptoms of shock are typically a weak, rapid **pulse**; cold, sweaty skin; and low **blood pressure**. The rapid pulse is the body's way of compensating for the low blood pressure. Treatment for bacteremic shock includes prompt antibiotic treatment and fluid replacement.

promptly with antibiotics and fluid replacement, can lead to **shock**, which has a high mortality rate of over 50%.

Abortion and Perinatal Infection

Campylobacter can cause inflammation of the placenta, which is the organ that unites the umbilical cord of the fetus to the uterus of the mother, resulting in insufficient transfer of

THE PLACENTA

The placenta is a spongy organ that develops inside the uterus of the mother during early pregnancy. At full term (before birth), the placenta stretches 5.9 to 7.9 inches (15 to 20 centimeters) across the uterus and is about 1.2 to 1.6 inches (3 to 4 centimeters) thick in the center, where the umbilical cord connects the fetus to the placenta. An average placenta weighs approximately 1.5 pounds (0.7 kilograms).

The placenta is a vascular organ, containing blood vessels from the fetus branching intricately and surrounded by maternal blood. The blood from the fetus and mother does not actually touch, but the placenta performs nutritive, respiratory, and excretory functions via exchange with the fetus's blood through the thin lining of the blood vessels.

Blood from the fetus enters the umbilical cord to the placenta. Through this intricate interlacing of blood vessels, nutrients and oxygen pass from the mother's side to the fetus's side and wastes and carbon dioxide pass from the fetus's side to the mother's. The placenta is responsible for the functions that the fetus's digestive system, lungs, and kidneys will be responsible for after birth. The placenta does provide a certain degree of protection against infectious agents, but can become infected and inflamed from organisms in the blood. Extra precautions that should be taken by expectant mothers to protect the fetus include avoiding the ingestion of raw foods, proper storage and handling of foods, and proper hygiene and sanitation measures.

oxygen, nutrients, and waste materials. This can eventually cause fetal death. The bacteria can also cross the placenta and infect the fetus. Why some pregnant women are affected and some are not remains unknown.

Reactive Arthritis (Reiter's Syndrome)

Arthritis can develop within 1 to 6 weeks after the onset of the bacterial infection. Apart from *Campylobacter*, other gastro-intestinal infectious agents such as *Salmonella* and *Shigella* also produce symptoms of reactive arthritis. The most common areas to be affected are the joints of the wrists, feet, ankles and knees, and the inflammation leads to stiffness, pain, swelling, warmth, and redness of the joints involved. Patients are usually treated with nonsteroidal anti-inflammatory drugs (NSAIDS) such as aspirin for the joint inflammation. Full recovery usually occurs, but the inflammation can last for weeks or months; for some patients, arthritic symptoms can persist for years.

The frequency of this complication depends on genetics. Patients who possess the gene for the human lymphocyte antigen B27 (HLA B27) have a higher predisposition for reactive arthritis. The majority of reactive arthritis patients, from 60–80%, have this gene.[9]

Guillain-Barré Syndrome

Guillain-Barré syndrome (GBS) is an autoimmune disorder, meaning that the body creates antibodies that attack its own tissue. In this case, the body targets specifically the myelin sheath lining of the nerves. The nerves themselves can be attacked as well. This attack causes an inflammatory reaction around the nerves and blocks the impulses and messages that are normally transported along the nerves. The disease first manifests as weakness, numbness, or tingling sensations in the limbs such as the hands and arms. Then, the illness progresses to a loss of motor function (paralysis), and finally affects the respiratory muscles, causing difficulty in breathing.

Most patients (80–85%) fully recover within weeks of the symptoms appearing, but a significant number of patients require mechanical ventilation (artificial breathing) and other medical intervention. If necessary, an intravenous (IV) line can be used to pass fluids into the patient's body. Nutrition can be given via a tube through the nose into the stomach. Recovery for these patients can take years, and some are left with severe neurological damage (paralysis). Approximately 2–5% of GBS cases result in death.[10]

It is estimated that GBS follows 0.1% of *Campylobacter* infections (1 GBS case per 1,000 campylobacteriosis cases). Approximately 40% of GBS patients have evidence of preceding campylobacteriosis, indicating *Campylobacter* as an important trigger. It seems that certain strains of *C. jejuni* are more likely to trigger GBS. The cell wall components of these strains have some regions that are similar to certain components associated with nerve cells, thus causing the immune system to become confused and attack its own cells. Of course, some people are more susceptible to this complication as well, but we do not yet know why.

5

How *Campylobacter* Organisms Cause Disease

Bacteria can be considered the dominant species on Earth because they have existed since prehistoric times. They exist in incalculable numbers and in all environments. With the discovery of fossils, bacteria have been traced back 3.5 billion years. With this in mind, it is no wonder that humans have a highly developed, complex immune system, which helps us stay healthy by fighting off invaders such as bacteria.

Before bacteria can harm us, they have to make contact with us and find a way to attach to and/or invade our cells, reproduce, and then cause damage while avoiding being killed by our immune system.

MAKING INITIAL CONTACT

Bacteria can make contact with us in three ways: ingestion, inhalation, and direct contact with the skin (Figure 5.1).

Ingestion

We can ingest bacteria, which is often the cause of food poisoning. Examples include eating leftovers that have spoiled, hamburgers that have not been cooked properly, and gravies that have not been reheated adequately. Food poisoning also results from eating foods that have become dangerous due to cross-contamination.

Food poisoning includes both infection and **intoxication**. Infection occurs when the bacteria grow and colonize the intestines and cause illness, such as is the case with *Campylobacter jejuni*. Intoxication occurs when the toxins that are produced and secreted by the bacteria in the

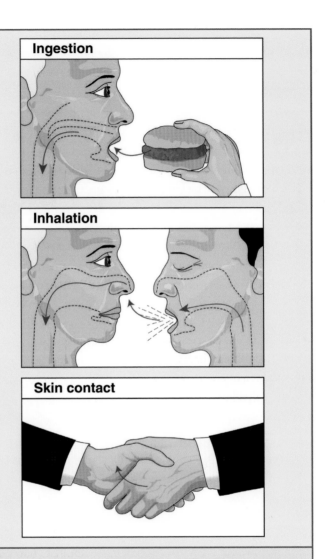

Figure 5.1 Bacteria must invade our body before they can cause harm. The three most frequent ways that we come in contact with bacteria is through ingestion (bacteria on or in food, or on our hands or utensils), inhalation (a person coughs or sneezes and you breathe in the bacteria), and skin contact (a person has bacteria on his or her hands and touches you or you touch an object that is coated with bacteria). These three methods are illustrated here.

intestine cause the symptoms of illness, such as in botulism. (For more information on botulism, see the box on pages 78–79.)

Inhalation

We can inhale the bacteria through a suspension of fine solid or liquid particles in gas (aerosols). For example, a farmer cleaning a barn with a high-pressure hose creates mist. This mist can contain bacteria that can be inhaled and then become a cause of disease. The bacteria can come from the feces of any of the animals that live in the barn. Keep in mind that these animals need not be ill or show any symptoms of illness in order to shed pathogens in their feces.

However, *Campylobacter* organisms are microaerophilic, too sensitive to air to survive in aerosols and, therefore, unless the farmer swallows some of the aerosols, is unlikely that *Campylobacter* will be transmitted in this fashion.

Contact With the Skin

We can come in contact with bacteria through our skin. Our skin, along with the mucosal linings of the respiratory, gastrointestinal, and genitourinary tracts, provides the first line of defense against pathogens. Our skin's protective characteristics include being dry and slightly acidic, having an adapted flora (bacteria that normally live on our skin without causing disease), and continuous shedding. Bacteria can more easily bypass the skin's defenses by entering through areas where our skin has been damaged, such as by puncture wounds or burns.

ATTACHMENT AND INVASION

Different bacteria have different mechanisms and characteristics that allow successful attachment and/or invasion of the body. For infection to occur, *Campylobacter* must first survive the low **pH** (acidic) conditions of the stomach and then colonize the small and large intestines. Successful colonization depends on *Campylobacter* being able to reach the cells that line the intestine, attach to them, and invade the body. The rapid darting motility of *Campylobacter*, due to the combination of their flagella and spiral shape, allows them to penetrate the viscous mucus layer to reach the epithelial cells, thereby allowing adherence and invasion.

Adherence and invasion of host cells are key factors of virulence for *C. jejuni*. The mechanisms involved in adherence and invasion are still vague, but are slowly becoming clearer. The processes of binding and entry of *C. jejuni* into epithelial cells and **macrophages,** scavengers of foreign invaders, are complex and involve a number of bacterial proteins and enzymes.

Recent studies indicate that *C. jejuni* contains a protein called CadF in the outer membrane of its cell wall that is required for binding to intestinal epithelial cells. This adherence enhances invasion.[11] Other proteins secreted by *C. jejuni*, such as Cia and Cjp29, have been found to be required for invasion.[12] Furthermore, studies indicate that at least 14 other proteins are synthesized upon incubation with mammalian cells in the laboratory.[13] Continued research will shed more light not only on how these proteins participate in successfully getting *C. jejuni* into the intestinal epithelial cells, but also on their degree of toxicity to the body.

Research has also indicated that *C. jejuni* can survive in macrophages, which are one of the natural defenders of the body that are supposed to kill foreign invaders. *C. jejuni* was found to be able to produce catalase, an enzyme that is able to deactivate the toxicity of hydrogen peroxide, which is released by macrophages to kill foreign invaders.[14] The importance of this research is that it indicates that *Campylobacter* may be "hiding" in our immune cells and using them for transportation. Reproduction occurs in the macrophages and death of the macrophages results in the spread of *Campylobacter*.

Only recently have we begun to understand *Campylobacter*. It is unknown how *Campylobacter* survives the low pH levels of the stomach, a natural defense mechanism of the digestive system. Many researchers and scientists are working with *Campylobacter* to understand the many aspects of the bacterium, such as why it

THE PH SCALE

The pH scale measures the acidity or alkalinity of solutions, represented by a quantitative scale (Figure 5.2). In chemistry, this is actually a measure of the concentration of the hydrogen ions. A higher concentration of hydrogen ions means a more acidic solution. Thus, lemon juice has more hydrogen ions than water.

The pH scale ranges from 0 to 14, with 7 representing a solution that is neither acidic nor basic. Thus, a solution with a pH of 7 such as pure water is considered neutral, whereas a solution with a pH of less than 7 is considered acidic and a solution with a pH greater than 7 is basic (alkaline). Each step down the scale represents a tenfold increase of hydrogen ions, which determines acidity. For example:

- Coffee has a pH of approximately 5, two steps below water (pH=7), indicating that coffee is 100 times more acidic than water.

- Orange juice has a pH of about 4 and so is 1,000 times more acidic than water and 10 times more acidic than coffee.

- Lemon juice, with a pH of 2, is 100 times more acidic than orange juice.

- The gastric juice in our stomach has a pH of approximately 1.5. As we eat, though, the food dilutes the gastric juice and increases the pH.

- Baking soda, which has a pH of 9, is 100 times *less* acidic than water and contains 100-fold fewer hydrogen ions.

is virulent, how it exerts its effects of virulence, and which strains are virulent, but a comprehensive understanding of the pathogenesis of *Campylobacter* is still elusive.

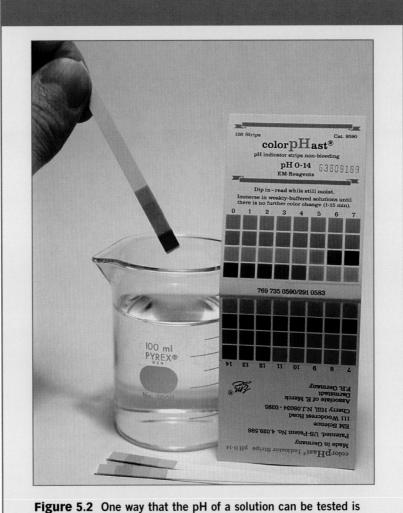

Figure 5.2 One way that the pH of a solution can be tested is by using commercially produced pH strips, such as the ones in this photo. The strip is dipped in the solution and changes color. The color can then be matched to a standardized marker that is provided with the test strips.

However, beginning in the late 1990s, some discoveries such as those mentioned above have shed light on the pathogenicity of *Campylobacter*. Recent technological advances in molecular microbiology are helping us answer the remaining questions.

REPRODUCTION

The goal of *Campylobacter*, once attached to and/or inside our epithelial cells after invasion, is to reproduce. Our intestinal tract supplies *Campylobacter* with the conditions that are

MOLECULAR GENETICS

Molecular microbiology is the study of the structures and processes of microbiological activities at the molecular level, including the study of proteins, nucleic acids (DNA), and **enzymes**, and how these molecules function and interact. In recent years, many molecular techniques have been developed or refined and are being used effectively to answer questions that previously could not be answered. Techniques include gene sequencing, in which the location of genes is mapped to specific chromosomes. This process provides knowledge of the gene structure and helps us begin to understand the gene function. Once we understand the specific gene function for a particular segment of DNA, such as producing a certain protein, scientists can associate these genes with specific characteristics of the organism.

As stated earlier, research has indicated that *Campylobacter* can survive in macrophages. Scientists have indicated this by cloning (making multiple identical copies) one strain that had a particular DNA fragment removed, whose function was to produce a catalase enzyme.[15] Hence, these clones were not able to produce the catalase enzyme. The function of catalase is to convert hydrogen peroxide to water and oxygen. Hydrogen peroxide is naturally produced by macrophages and contributes to their ability to kill invaders. The scientists then incubated these required, including warmth, moisture, nutrients, and low oxygen and acid levels. The newly divided cells seek out more epithelial cells and more opportunities to replicate.

As the number of *Campylobacter* organisms increases, so do the waste products and toxins excreted by these organisms. The higher the virulence of the infecting *Campylobacter* strain and the higher the numbers of *Campylobacter* in the body, the graver the degree of abdominal pain and diarrhea will be. Diarrhea occurs when the intestinal tract is unable to absorb nutrients due to tissue damage; undigested food,

clones of *Campylobacter* bacteria that are unable to inactivate hydrogen peroxide with macrophage cells (grown in the laboratory) and found that these isolates, compared to the non-mutated original *Campylobacter*, could not survive in the macrophages for 72 hours. As well, in piglets, the original strain caused lesions in the intestinal tract whereas the mutant strain did not (piglets are often used in these experiments because their digestive system is very similar to that of humans). This indicates that catalase production is an important part of *Campylobacter* survival.

Molecular genetics are also used in many aspects of medicine and in our everyday lives. Recombinant DNA techniques, such as combining DNA fragments from two different sources, have allowed scientists to create bacteria that can produce human insulin, a critical hormone required by people with diabetes. Another example is human growth hormone, produced by bacteria, that allows many children who are deficient of human growth hormone to be able to obtain this once rare hormone from reliable suppliers.

Many of the foods that we eat are genetically modified. Foreign or modified DNA is commonly inserted into plants to enhance or bring about certain desired traits, such as sweeter red peppers, strawberries that resist frost, tomatoes that ripen more slowly, and virus-resistant potatoes.

unabsorbed water, dead cells, and waste products are flushed out. Grossly bloody diarrhea is seen when considerable damage has been done to the intestinal tract, causing lesions in the inflamed mucosa, which leads to bleeding. Damage to our intestinal tract by the invasion of *Campylobacter*, which the body recognizes as a foreign invader, sets off our immune system.

LINES OF DEFENSE IN OUR IMMUNE SYSTEM

Humans have a complex immune system capable of recognizing and defending against foreign organisms. Any foreign organism, including infectious agents or substances such as snake venom or chemicals, is called an **antigen**. Antigens stimulate an immune response by activating the **lymphocytes** of the **lymphoid system**. The lymphoid system is a subsystem of the circulatory system responsible for fluid balance and drainage. It also produces lymphocytes, a type of white blood cell (also commonly called leukocytes) that fights antigens such as *C. jejuni*.

Defenses such as lymphocytes keep our blood and tissues free of foreign agents. Lymphocytes are part of the body's **specific defense system**, which responds to specific threats by infectious agents such as bacteria. This system includes lymphocytes such as **B cells**, which create fighter antibodies, and **T cells.**

Our bodies also have a **nonspecific defense system**, which fights all foreign bodies the same way. These defenses include:

- Skin barrier

- Natural defenses of the intestinal tract

- Inflammation process

- The **complement system**, which involves activation of a cascade of over 30 proteins secreted by liver cells and macrophages to ultimately result in complement protein C3b adhering to the surface of invaders, thus acting as an indicator to aid in **phagocytosis**

- Phagocytosis, which is ingestion or engulfment of foreign invaders by white blood cells or leukocytes such as neutrophils and macrophages, commonly called **phagocytes**.

Skin Barrier

Our skin provides the first line of defense against pathogens. It protects us from invading bacteria by:

- Being dry and slightly acidic, thus an uninviting environment for most foreign bacteria

- Continuously shedding, so if other bacteria are able to attach to our skin, they are rapidly shed along with the dead skin cells (Figure 5.3)

- Having an adapted flora (bacteria that normally live on our skin without causing disease). The bacteria that normally reside on our skin are Gram-positive. These bacteria are able to adapt to the dry, acidic environment better than Gram-negative bacteria because of the peptidoglycan in their cell wall structure. These bacteria give us protection by **competitive exclusion**: When species compete for the same ecological niche, one species survives and thrives and the other dies or must find another niche.

Natural Defenses of the Intestinal Tract

Our intestinal tract (Figure 5.4) is exposed to many microbes through the foods that we eat. It has its own natural defenses to deal with these organisms. For example, mucus, which is secreted continuously, provides protection by trapping bacteria.

The mucus, along with bacteria, food, and water, is moved along by **peristalsis** (wave-like contractions) that occurs in the esophagus, stomach, and intestines. The primary function of peristalsis is to move food to the stomach, help mix and distribute the food's nutrients throughout the intestines

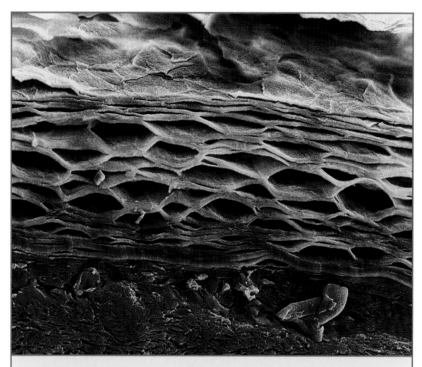

Figure 5.3 The skin is our first line of defense against invading microorganisms. Not only is it dry and acidic, and thus inhospitable for most bacteria, but skin cells are continuously shedding. When skin cells are shed, any bacteria on the skin will also be removed. A cross-section of skin cells is shown in this photomicrograph. Notice the shedding of the top layer.

so the nutrients make contact with the epithelial cells for absorption, and move wastes out of the body.

Bacterial growth is controlled mechanically by peristalsis since these waves dislodge bacteria from the digestive tract. In addition, cells in the intestine grow and are replaced every 3 to 5 days; this natural sloughing off of cells also provides protection against infection.

Another defense mechanism of the intestinal tract is **bile salts** that are secreted by the gallbladder into the **duodenum**, the first part of the small intestine, to help digest fat. Bile salts

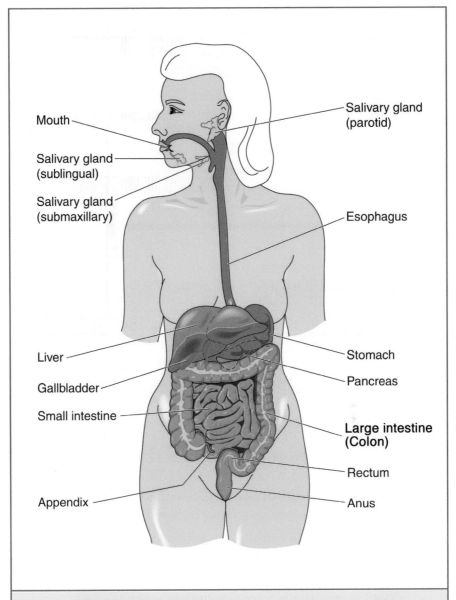

Figure 5.4 The digestive tract, illustrated here, also provides defenses against bacteria. Mucus traps bacteria in the mouth and esophagus, the stomach acid kills many bacteria, and bile salts in the duodenum interfere with bacterial attachment.

aid in the digestion of fats by separating the larger fats into tinier and tinier droplets, similar to how detergent or dish-washing liquid disperses fat into tiny droplets. This detergent effect interferes with the invasion and adherence of bacteria.

Most of the bile salts are reabsorbed in the lower small intes-tine and recycled for use again. However, if the intestinal tract is damaged, reabsorption is impaired and the bile salts move into the large intestine, where they interfere with the absorption of water and sodium, thus contributing to watery diarrhea.

The resident microflora that normally inhabit the intes-tinal tract also aid in protection against bacteria. The microflora compete for resources with invading bacteria. Some resident bacteria can make and secrete antibacterial products to deter the incoming bacteria. In addition, the oxygen level of the intestinal tract is very low since 97% of resident microflora are strict **anaerobes**, requiring no oxygen. The atmosphere of our intestinal tract is mostly anaerobic, with tiny pockets of air containing little oxygen. Aerobic bacteria, which require oxygen, have great difficulty competing with these anaerobes. *Campylobacter* are microaerophilic, so they are able to survive in the small pockets of the intestine that contain some oxygen.

ONCE INFECTION HAS OCCURRED

For any pathogenic bacteria to be successful, they must overcome all of these natural defenses. Not all strains of *Campylobacter* are virulent. The ones that are virulent, however, must be able to survive the acidic conditions of the stomach once ingested, adhere to and/or invade the epithelial cells, and reproduce. Both the nonspecific and specific defense systems are stimulated by exposure to *Campylobacter*.

Inflammation

Reproduction of *Campylobacter* damages the epithelial cells, causing inflammation. Inflammation serves to localize and eliminate the harmful agent, remove damaged tissue, and begin the process of healing and repair. The four signs of inflammation are redness, warmth, swelling, and pain. Think of the last time you injured yourself, whether it was a cut on your hand or a scrape on your knee. The injured area likely felt warm, looked red and swollen, and felt painful. The same processes occur in your damaged intestinal tract.

The redness and warmth are due to the dilation of blood vessels, which allows more blood to flow into the damaged area. The blood carries white blood cells such as phagocytes and certain proteins that fight the foreign bacteria. These cells and proteins travel through the permeable blood vessel lining into the tissues, thus causing the swelling. The pain is due to the changes in the tissues.

Throughout this process, chemicals released from our defense system mediate these **vascular** and **cellular** changes. Fever results when inflammation is serious and significant amounts of these chemicals have been released to affect the hypothalamus, which is the part of the brain that regulates body temperature. More and more of our defensive cells are called upon until we either win the war or lose, in which case **bacteremic shock** ensues.

Activation of the Complement System

The complement system can be activated by molecules in the surface membranes of invaders or by antibodies produced by B cells bound to the invading organisms. Hence, it works with both the nonspecific and specific defenses of the body. This complex system of more than 30 proteins secreted by the liver normally circulates inactivated in the blood. Once activated, a chain reaction occurs whereby one complement protein activates the next complement protein and so on. Ultimately, the result is a process called **opsonization**, where the complement protein C3b adheres to the surface of invaders. This aids phagocytosis by phagocytes because the phagocytes are able to recognize the C3b molecule. After engulfment, the invader is killed by digestive enzymes present in the phagocytes.

Leukocytes

We naturally have **white blood cells** (also called leukocytes) in the blood, on the order of 5,000 to 10,000 per cubic millimeter of blood (approximately the volume of a tiny droplet of blood from a small pin prick). They are called white blood cells because they do not have **hemoglobin**, the red, iron-rich protein that binds oxygen in the red blood cells.

Leukocytes are grouped into 3 major classes: granulocytes, monocytes, and lymphocytes (Figure 5.5). Granulocytes and monocytes are scavenger cells that are part of the nonspecific defense system, while lymphocytes are part of the body's specific defense system.

Granulocytes, of which neutrophils are the most common, are the first to arrive at an injured site (within an hour) to engulf and kill invading organisms via the process called phagocytosis. Phagocytosis involves engulfment of the invading organism by the white blood cell (phagocyte), which then secretes digestive enzymes to kill it.

Monocytes circulate in the blood and mature into macrophages, which tend to settle into tissues such as in the lymphoid tissues, liver, and intestinal cells. Macrophages are different from neutrophils in that they arrive much later at the injured site, live longer, and are much larger. Unlike neutrophils, after phagocytosis of *Campylobacter*, macrophages can present portions of the organism on their cell membrane, thus being antigen-presenting cells and aiding in activating the lymphocytes. Both neutrophils and macrophages are drawn toward an injured site by substances given off by the bacteria or infected area, or due to signaling of the complement system.

Lymphocytes are another type of white blood cell that circulates in the blood vessels. They are unique in that they are

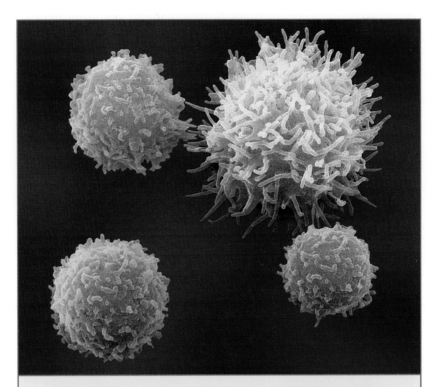

Figure 5.5 Lymphocytes and monocytes, shown here, are types of white blood cells. White blood cells act to protect the body from foreign microorganisms. In this photo, the monocyte is the larger cell.

also concentrated in lymphoid organs and tissues, such as the spleen, thymus, lymph nodes, and in between the intestinal epithelial cells. They circulate in an immature form until activated by antigens.

There are two kinds of lymphocytes: the T cells and the B cells. Both types have **receptor** molecules on their surfaces that allow them to bind to specific antigens. *Campylobacter*, being an antigen, has regions on its cell wall surfaces that fit and bind to the receptor molecules of lymphocytes. Upon binding with the bacteria, the B cells are stimulated to multiply and produce numerous antibodies to target and destroy *Campylobacter*. T cells are activated to target and destroy cells that have been infected by *Campylobacter*, such as macrophages that have ingested *Campylobacter* and are displaying parts of *Campylobacter*'s components on their own cell wall.

B cells are also called memory cells because they remember previous antigens. Thus, if the same antigen is encountered in the future, the immune system will react much faster and with more vigor to fight that antigen. To illustrate, people who contract campylobacteriosis in childhood and then are repeatedly exposed to the same bacteria experience subsequent bouts of campylobacteriosis that are less severe and of shorter duration as they get older.

However, bacteria are able to adapt quickly to the threats posed by our immune systems. These single-celled organisms are capable of rapid genetic changes, changing the composition of their cell membranes so the B cells cannot recognize them. The immune system must start its fight against the antigen anew. This is one example of how bacteria can avoid the host's immune defenses. This variability of surface antigenic regions is also important in determining the severity of the infection. Certain strains of *C. jejuni* have regions that are closely matched with structures of our nerve cells and, hence, upon stimulation of the immune system, huge numbers of our defenders end up attacking our nerve cells, believing that they are antigens. This results in Guillain-Barré syndrome.

In mild infections, there are adequate white blood cells in the blood to fight, ingest, and kill the invaders. In moderate to serious infections, enormous numbers of white blood cells are produced (prompted by the chemical factors) and sent to the site of injury to fight until there are no longer any invaders. After the fight, all the dead cells (foreign bacteria as well as our body's own defensive cells) are cleared from the blood and tissues in the form of pus. The area repairs and heals itself by regenerating the lost cells through new tissue formation. In serious cases, the body is not able to repair itself and the result is chronic disease or death.

In summary, *Campylobacter* causes disease by invading and adhering to our intestinal epithelial cells, and by reproducing and causing damage to those cells. Infection causes our immune system to respond. Inflammation occurs, our complement proteins are activated, our phagocytes are called upon, and our specific defense system is set into motion. The exact mechanisms by which *Campylobacter* adheres, invades, and causes damage are unclear, but many researchers are experimenting with *Campylobacter* to find answers. Research suggests that *Campylobacter* can survive in macrophages, thus "hiding" in our own cells. Different strains of *Campylobacter* also invade the body in different ways. Also, recall that the strength of each individual's immune system will influence the outcome of disease. Every infectious agent needs to make initial contact with the body, enter it, and find a place to reproduce. There are numerous ways that this can occur. Not all bacteria have flagella, nor do they all have the ability to adhere and invade. Some can adhere but not invade. Some invade and are able to move from one epithelial cell to another. Some are able to change their antigenic regions continuously and rapidly. Others can secrete fatal toxins or form spores. The ways in which bacteria create disease are many and this is something to keep in mind when studying them.

6

Campylobacter in the Food and Water

Although the reservoirs of *Campylobacter* are many and include animals such as cattle, dogs, cats, wild birds, chickens, and turkeys, *Campylobacter* infections are mainly associated with food. There have been cases of *Campylobacter* infections arising from contact with pets and from caretakers of infants or children infected with *Campylobacter*, but the fact remains that campylobacteriosis is primarily a disease of food poisoning. In the food supply, the main sources of *Campylobacter* infections are poultry, unpasteurized milk, and untreated water.

In the United States, agricultural practices have undergone a gigantic transformation in the last 30 years. Many advances in science and technology allowed these changes to be implemented. We have gone from the backyard farm that used to be a family enterprise to huge factory farms that are fully automated in terms of feeding, waste removal, slaughtering, and packaging.

REGULATING THE POULTRY INDUSTRY

This change is very evident in the poultry industry. Since many *Campylobacter* infections are associated with poultry, it is important to take measures to control the transmission of the bacteria during poultry processing (Figure 6.1). Transmission of *Campylobacter* can occur at any point in the process of hatching, growing, slaughtering, processing, distributing, or preparing chicken for a meal. Like other foods, poultry goes through numerous steps before reaching our plates at home or in a restaurant. When reading about the steps below, think of

70

Figure 6.1 *Campylobacter* is often present on the skin of chickens, and thus, can be transmitted through the processing, cooking, and consumption of poultry. Shown here is an image of chicken skin under a microscope. *Campylobacter* cells are stained fluorescent green.

all the chances for cross-contamination. Remember that these are factory farms, capable of processing more than 90,000 chickens each day.

1. Fertilized eggs are placed in poultry incubators to keep warm and to be turned and rotated automatically until ready to hatch. Large commercial incubators can hold tens of thousands of eggs at one time.

2. Upon hatching, automated factory poultry farms with computerized feed bins, automated water delivery, and automated waste removal provide the nutrition required for the chickens to grow to full size, with each chicken usually individually caged. Most broiler chickens are ready for market by 7 weeks of age.

3. When the appropriate weight is reached at approximately 7 weeks of age, the birds are slaughtered for their meat. The birds are transported in cages to the slaughterhouse, where they are removed from the cages. Their feet are attached to moving shackles where they are suspended in the air upside down and their throats are slit with a knife that has an electric current running through it. Hence, the chickens are stunned at the same time as their throats are slit, thereby killing them instantly and more humanely. The chickens are then bled, scalded in hot water tanks to soften the skin, and defeathered via a sequence of feather-picking machines that remove different sets of feathers. The heads are then pulled off and the legs removed mechanically. The carcasses drop and are rehung by their hocks (joints) prior to entering the evisceration line.

4. Fully automated evisceration is performed to remove the internal organs.

5. The carcass and the internal organs are inspected after evisceration. In the United States, inspectors from the U.S. Department of Agriculture (USDA) carry out this inspection. Carcasses or parts of carcasses that do not pass inspection are removed.

6. The approved carcasses are then cleaned and visceral organs are separated.

7. After washing, the carcasses are chilled. Water chilling is the method used in the United States (as opposed to air chilling in Europe) and includes overflows of water in huge tanks to decrease the temperature of the carcasses. This process is very water intensive. The birds are then cut into various pieces and packaged on plastic foam trays covered with a plastic film as normally seen at supermarkets.

8. A final chill is performed and the final temperature reached prior to shipment is just above the freezing point for poultry, approximately 28° to 30°F (-2° to -1°C). After slaughter, the fresh meat of the poultry should be consumed within 2 to 3 weeks or frozen.

9. If frozen commercially, various flavorings, salts, or oils may be injected into the poultry to increase the juiciness or tenderness of the meat. The injections are automated and the label on the package will include the added ingredients along with instructions for safe handling. Most chicken is sold fresh and most turkey is sold frozen.

10. The poultry may also be processed into other products. Examples include breaded or battered poultry such as chicken nuggets or marinated poultry with flavors such as teriyaki. The numbers of processed poultry products are vast and steadily increasing because poultry is relatively low in cost compared to other meats. The application of the factory farm and assembly-line-type slaughtering, evisceration, and inspection has decreased the cost of chicken tremendously in the last 30 years.

Poultry is an excellent growth medium for bacteria, not only for *Campylobacter*, but also for other bacteria such as *Salmonella*, *Staphylococcus*, and *Listeria*. Because of the numerous steps involved in poultry processing and the sheer volume of chickens processed, the USDA has set careful regulation and monitoring guidelines for these processes. Poultry contamination usually occurs when the carcasses come into contact with parts of the body that are high in bacteria, such as the intestines. The feathers also usually have high numbers of bacteria due to contact with feces. Therefore, the defeathering area is, by law, required to be separated by a wall from the evisceration area to avoid cross-contamination.

After evisceration, the carcasses must be washed before chilling. During water chilling, a specified amount of overflow for each tank is required. Though this process uses a lot of water, it is important to dilute the bacteria that are washed off to minimize contamination.

Another important factor in limiting contamination is controlling the temperature of the poultry carcasses. Temperature is an important regulator of microbial growth. As with all bacteria, *Campylobacter* are unicellular and multiply by cell division, where 1 cell becomes 2 identical organisms, then the 2 becomes 4, then 4 becomes 8, and so forth until there are billions. When optimal conditions are present, the average doubling time for many bacteria is 20 minutes. At this rate, a single bacterium can produce approximately 70 billion cells in 12 hours!

Temperature influences the rate of microbial growth, along with the availability of nutrients, water or moisture, pH (acidic or nonacidic), oxygen levels, and, of course, the innate ability of the species to multiply. *Campylobacter* prefers a temperature between 86° and 113°F (30°C to 45°C), so chilling limits its growth. *Salmonella*, on the other hand, can grow in temperatures ranging from 41.4° to 115.2°F (5.2° to 46.2°C). Therefore, the carcasses must be chilled to 28° to 30°F (-2° to -1°C) prior to shipping in refrigerated trucks as temperature is critical in controlling pathogenic bacterial growth.

Lowering the temperature controls the growth rate, but increasing the temperature high enough will destroy the pathogenic bacteria. Processed poultry products such as chicken nuggets much reach internal temperatures that are adequate to kill the bacteria before the product is frozen.

When raw or cooked products are packaged, workers must follow strict hygiene and sanitary procedures, such as wearing disposable gloves, hairnets, and uniforms. The trucks utilized must be cleaned and sanitized frequently, just as all transporting cages, processing equipment, and floors are cleaned and sanitized to reduce the chance of cross-contamination. *Campylobacter* has been reported as being transmitted by cages, by workers (from feces on their boots), and from improperly cleaned equipment.

PRESERVING FOODS

Various methods of preservation are employed to prevent food from spoiling after harvest or slaughter. This includes chilling or refrigeration, freezing, drying or dehydration, salting, canning, acidification (as with pickling using vinegar), irradiation, the addition of antimicrobials or chemicals such as sodium nitrate, and pasteurization. Preservation works by either limiting or controlling one of the key factors required for microbial growth. Examples include limiting warmth or moisture or by manipulating the environment in such a manner that the bacteria have a difficult time replicating.

Chilling or Refrigeration

Chilling or refrigeration will increase the life of most foods, including poultry. Animal meat spoils rapidly at room temperature as bacteria use the nutrients, multiply, and produce waste products. Chilling slows down this growth and allows foods to last longer. Poultry stored in home refrigerators should be used within three days to ensure freshness and safety, as *Campylobacter* will survive refrigerator temperatures.

Freezing

Freezing occurs when the temperature is low enough to convert the water in the food into ice. This process will further slow down or inhibit bacterial growth or spoilage. Freezing will kill some pathogens, but not *Campylobacter*.

When stored in the freezer, poultry should be used within three months. Note that the temperature required for freezing foods is lower than the temperature required for freezing water because the water in foods contains solutes that lower the freezing point by making it harder for the water molecules to arrange themselves neatly into a lattice formation. This is why the freezing point of poultry is approximately 26°F (−3.3°C) but the freezing point of pure water is 32°F (0°C).

Drying or Dehydration

Drying or dehydration is not used for poultry, but is used for other meats such as beef. Dehydration works by removing the water that bacteria require for growth. *Campylobacter* is extremely sensitive to drying and without moisture, will be unable to live. Thus, drying a food is an effective way to kill *Campylobacter*.

Salting

Salting, used to preserve fish, or adding sugar to preserve fruit also works by removing the water that bacteria require for growth. Water is taken up by the salt or sugar, making it unavailable for use by the bacteria.

Canning

If food is heated to the appropriate temperature for the correct amount of time while sealed in an airtight container, that food will remain free of bacterial growth until it is opened. In this process, cans are filled with food, the air is forced out to create a vacuum, and then the can is sealed and sterilized. The temperature and the heating time required to kill all the microorganisms, including *Campylobacter*, vary with the food being processed and the size of the container. Poultry products are often canned, such as for chicken noodle soups and canned chicken meat.

Acidification

Acidification of foods with vinegar (acetic acid) or other acids including benzoic or propionic acids retard the growth of microorganisms simply because many organisms cannot grow in acidic conditions. Along with the other growth requirements, *Campylobacter* prefers pH levels of 4.9 to 9.5. To inhibit the growth of *Campylobacter* and other bacteria, the food can be acidified.

Irradiation

Irradiation has been approved for controlling bacteria in raw chicken and turkey since 1992, although there have been many misconceptions regarding its safety. Some states have prohibited the use of irradiation due to consumer resistance and fear of the process. Irradiation involves exposing foods to specified levels of radiation such as gamma rays for specified periods of time to control and destroy microorganisms by damaging their genetic material. Affected bacteria will be unable to survive or multiply. Both *Campylobacter* and *Salmonella* are sensitive to irradiation.

Irradiation does not make food radioactive, since no radioactive material is added to the food. Thus, there is no danger to humans except for workers who do not take precautions when they irradiate the foods. This method is also used to sterilize many medical devices, which also does not expose humans to radiation.

The maximum radiation dose set for poultry is 3 kiloGrays (kGy). Packages of poultry that have been treated with irradiation must be labeled with the international radura symbol along with the statement, "treated with irradiation" or "treated by irradiation" (Figure 6.2). Poultry that have been irradiated can still be cross-contaminated with pathogenic bacteria, such as from contaminated poultry.

Antimicrobials

Antimicrobials include many agents that prevent the growth of molds, yeasts, and bacteria. One common antimicrobial used in luncheon meats, ham, and bacon is sodium nitrate, used during the curing of the meats to prevent the growth of bacteria, mainly *Clostridium botulinum*, which causes botulism. The addition of sodium nitrate as a preservative is controversial because people who consume sodium nitrate produce compounds known as nitrosamines, which are carcinogenic.

BOTULISM FROM CANNED FOODS

Commercially canned foods are extremely safe, especially with today's strict regulations. Home canning, on the other hand, has resulted in some cases of botulism, which is a serious paralytic illness caused by the neurotoxin (nerve toxin) produced by *Clostridium botulinum*, a Gram-positive, anaerobic, spore-forming bacteria. There are three kinds of botulism. The most common kind is infant botulism (72%) that occurs when infants consume the spores of *Clostridium botulinum*, which can be found in honey. The second type is ingestion of foods contaminated with *Clostridium botulinum* (25%). The third kind is wound botulism (3%), caused by toxins produced from a wound that has been infected with *Clostridium botulinum*. Although wound botulism is rare, there have been increases in California among those who inject black-tar heroin, causing infections at the injection site. Wound botulism can be prevented with prompt medical care. An antitoxin, if administered early, can reduce the symptoms and prevent irreversible nerve damage.

Approximately 110 botulism cases are reported each year in the United States. *Clostridium botulinum* spores are commonly found in soil. They are rod-shaped organisms that grow into vegetative cells that produce toxins in anaerobic conditions, such as those created in home canning. These spores can remain harmless in soils and water for many years until they are supplied with optimal conditions, including moisture, warmth, and very low to no oxygen.

By law, the USDA limits the amount of sodium nitrate that can legally be added to these foods.

Pasteurization

Pasteurization, as explained in the box entitled "Outbreak of *C. jejuni* Infections in Wisconsin, 2001" in Chapter 3, is the

Classic symptoms of botulism among adults include blurred and double vision, slurred speech, difficulty swallowing, and muscle weakness leading to paralysis of the arms, legs, trunk, and respiratory muscles. The bacterial toxin also attacks the nerves. Eventually, the nerves will no longer be able to transmit messages, thus resulting in paralysis. For infants, the disease begins with constipation and lethargy, leading to poor muscle tone and paralysis.

Outbreaks have occurred from some unusual sources, such as unrefrigerated chopped garlic in oil, chili peppers, home-canned or fermented fish, and improperly handled baked potatoes wrapped in aluminum foil. Strict hygienic procedures such as refrigeration, keeping foods hot until served, and proper sterilization and handling during canning will prevent such outbreaks. The botulism toxin is destroyed by heat, so individuals eating home-canned foods should boil the food for 10 minutes.

Ingestion of spores (rather than the active bacteria) normally is not sufficient to cause botulism in infants over one year of age and in adults. Although the spores may germinate into vegetative cells, they are unable to compete with the normal flora present in mature intestines. Infants under one year of age have underdeveloped flora. Thus, young infants should not be fed honey because honey contains spores of *Clostridium botulinum*, which will colonize the intestinal tract and produce the neurotoxin.

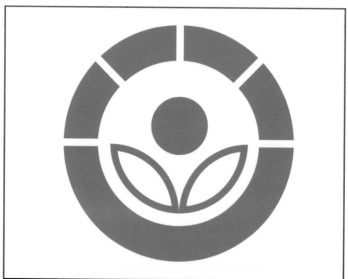

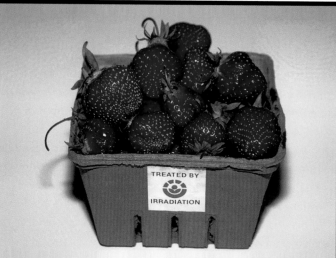

Figure 6.2 Some foods, such as meat, poultry, and certain fruits, are treated with radiation. This process, called irradiation, kills bacteria such as *Campylobacter* and *Salmonella*. Foods treated with irradiation are marked with the radura symbol (top) and are marked with the words "treated by irradiation," as seen on the package of strawberries in the bottom photograph.

partial sterilization of a substance without significantly altering the chemical composition. Milk and juice are pasteurized to destroy pathogenic microorganisms. Pasteurization involves heating the substance to high temperatures for specified amounts of time. Pasteurization is different from sterilization, which renders a product sterile, indicating that there is a complete absence of microorganisms rather than a reduction in numbers of bacteria. This is why milk and juice still require refrigeration or else spoilage will occur rapidly. *Campylobacter* has been found in unpasteurized milk.

PROTECTING THE WATER SUPPLY

The water we drink, cook with, and wash with is another major source of *Campylobacter*. Water that is provided by municipalities has been filtered and treated before it reaches our faucets. Treatment of all drinking water by the appropriate agencies and universal pasteurization of all milk products would eliminate the majority of outbreaks associated with *Campylobacter*. The next chapter deals with how we, as consumers and individuals, can prevent *Campylobacter* infections.

7

What Can You Do to Prevent Campylobacteriosis?

"I wonder if I ate something that just did not agree with me," or "It must be something I ate," are common statements by many people after a few bouts of acute diarrhea. It is no doubt that the food supply in the United States is one of the safest in the world, especially since the advent of modern technologies to preserve foods and detect contamination. However, when huge volumes of food such as broiler chickens are produced, as described in Chapter 6, and so many microorganisms are awaiting opportunities to enter a welcoming environment and replicate, it is no wonder that there are so many cases of foodborne illnesses. The CDC estimates that foodborne diseases caused by bacteria, viruses, parasites, toxins, and metals result in approximately 76 million illnesses, 325,000 hospitalizations, and 5,000 deaths in the United States annually.[16]

With so many foodborne illnesses, it is difficult to find people who have not been afflicted by foodborne illness themselves or at least known someone who has suffered from foodborne illness. Government agencies have made food safety a high priority, but consumers must accept their share of responsibility after they bring food home from the supermarket. Many foodborne illnesses can be prevented. The safety practices outlined in this chapter are beneficial for preventing foodborne illnesses from many agents, not just *Campylobacter*.

Remember: There are many pathogens in many foods other than poultry. Food safety basics should always be followed to prevent foodborne illness.

The following prevention tips are provided by the U.S. Food and Drug Administration (FDA), which has put together a fact sheet entitled "The Unwelcome Dinner Guest: Preventing Foodborne Illness." This information is available online at *http://www.cfsan.fda.gov/~dms/fdunwelc.html*. The FDA is the federal agency responsible for promoting and protecting public health.

PREVENTING FOODBORNE ILLNESS
At the Supermarket

While shopping for groceries, pay attention to the foods that you are choosing and the order in which you go through the store.

THE U.S. FOOD AND DRUG ADMINISTRATION (FDA)

The U.S. Food and Drug Administration (FDA) is responsible for promoting and protecting public health. The FDA achieves these goals by ensuring that safe and effective products reach the market in a timely manner and by monitoring products for their continued safety after they are in use.

More than 9,000 staff members at the FDA in 167 field offices focus on inspection and surveillance, laboratory work, and public and industry education. Consumer protection is the overall goal. This includes promoting safer food handling practices, ensuring a safe blood supply, approving new drugs, and regulating and approving varied products such as food additives, medical and surgical devices, radiation-emitting consumer products (e.g., cell phones and microwaves), and animal drugs.

- Pick up packaged and canned foods first. Avoid bulging, dented, or cracked containers and lids.

- Purchase only pasteurized milk and cheeses, and pasteurized or otherwise treated ciders and juices. Remember that outbreaks of campylobacteriosis have occurred with unpasteurized milk. Pay attention to the expiration date, as pasteurization does not mean sterilization.

- Select frozen foods and perishables such as poultry, meat, or fish last. Put these products in separate plastic bags so that drippings (such as poultry drippings) do not contaminate other foods in your cart such as lettuce. For fresh meats such as poultry, pay attention to the package date.

- Do not purchase any packages that are open, torn, or crushed. When choosing frozen packages, choose those that are below the frost line in the store's freezer.

- Check for cleanliness at the meat or fish counter and at the salad counter, where cross-contamination can easily occur.

- Take an ice chest along to keep frozen and perishable foods cold if it will take longer than one hour to get home, especially in the summer, as *Campylobacter* can grow at room temperature and above.

At Home

Upon reaching home, store the food properly (Figure 7.1).

- Refrigerate and freeze perishables immediately. The refrigerator temperature should be 40°F (5°C) and the freezer should be 0°F (-18°C). Invest in a refrigerator and freezer thermometer. *Campylobacter* can still survive in refrigerators although refrigeration will retard its growth.

- Poultry and meat to be refrigerated may be stored as purchased in the original plastic wrap for 1 to 2 days.

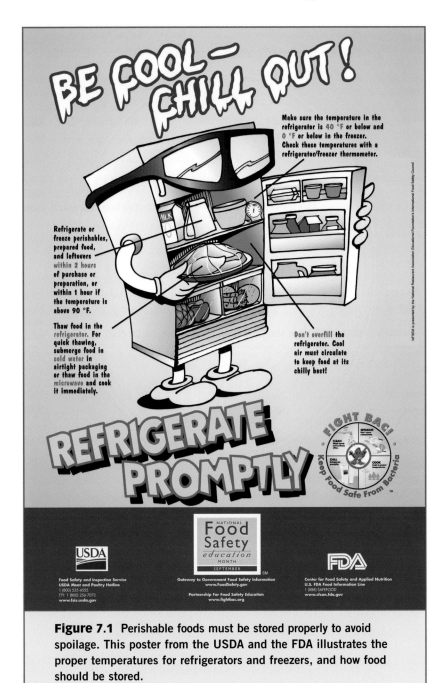

Figure 7.1 Perishable foods must be stored properly to avoid spoilage. This poster from the USDA and the FDA illustrates the proper temperatures for refrigerators and freezers, and how food should be stored.

(See Table 7.1: "How Long Will It Keep?") Otherwise, freeze it. Although freezing will not completely kill *Campylobacter*, it will decrease the numbers by killing some.

- If only part of the meat or poultry is going to be used right away, separate the portions in a hygienic manner (see "Keep It Clean," below), place them in sealed containers, and label the portions with the date. Make sure that the juices cannot escape the container to contaminate other foods.

- Foods to be frozen should be wrapped tightly or placed in freezer bags. Leftovers should be stored in sealed containers.

- Do not crowd the refrigerator or freezer so tightly that air cannot circulate. Check the leftovers in covered dishes and storage bags daily for spoilage. Anything that looks or smells suspicious should be thrown out. Do not take any chances if you cannot remember how long the food has been in there.

- Always check the labels on cans or jars to determine how the contents should be stored. Many items besides fresh meats, vegetables, and dairy products need to be kept cold. For instance, mayonnaise and ketchup should be stored in the refrigerator after opening. If you have neglected to refrigerate items that should be refrigerated, it is best to throw them out.

Keep It Clean

When preparing food, the number one rule is to keep everything clean, including the surfaces that the food comes into contact with and the people handling the food. Many cases of campylobacteriosis have been due to poor sanitation.

- Wash hands with warm water and soap for at least 20 seconds before starting to prepare a meal and especially

Table 7.1 – How Long Will It Keep?

The following table is taken from "The Unwelcome Dinner Guest: Preventing Foodborne Illness" at http://www.cfsan.fda.gov/~dms/fdunwelc.html. It provides a list of storage guidelines for some of the foods that are regularly served on our dinner tables.

Product	Storage Period	
	In Refrigerator 40°F (5°C)	In Freezer 0°F (-18°C)
Fresh Meat		
Ground beef	1-2 days	3-4 months
Steaks and roasts	3-5 days	6-12 months
Pork		
Chops	3-5 days	4-6 months
Ground	1-2 days	3-4 months
Roasts	3-5 days	4-6 months
Cured meats		
Lunch meat	3-5 days	1-2 months
Sausage	1-2 days	1-2 months
Gravy	1-2 days	2-3 months
Fish		
Lean (such as cod, flounder, haddock)	1-2 days	up to 6 months
Fatty (such as blue, perch, salmon)	1-2 days	2-3 months
Chicken		
Whole	1-2 days	12 months
Parts	1-2 days	9 months
Giblets	1-2 days	3-4 months
Dairy Products		
Swiss, brick, processed cheese	3-4 weeks	*
Milk	5 days	1 month
Ice cream, ice milk	-	2-4 months
Eggs		
Fresh in shell	3 weeks	-
Hard-boiled	1 week	-

* Cheese can be frozen, but freezing will affect the texture and taste.
Sources: Food Marketing Institute for fish and dairy products, USDA for all other foods.

after handling raw meat or poultry. Use at least a dime-sized amount of soap and rub hands together vigorously.

- If you have long hair, pull it back into a ponytail or use bobby pins to keep hair off your face.

- Be sure that any open sores or cuts on the hands are completely covered. If the sore or cut is infected, do not cook.

- Avoid touching your face and hair when preparing food.

- Keep the work area clean and uncluttered. Wash countertops with a solution of 1 teaspoon chlorine bleach to 1 quart water or with a commercial kitchen-cleaning agent diluted according to product directions. It is a good idea to keep a spray bottle that has a dilution of 1 teaspoon of chlorine bleach to 1 quart of water by the sink to use for sanitizing. Be careful not to spray any on your clothes. *Campylobacter,* as well as many other infectious agents, cannot survive bleaching.

- Keep dishcloths, brushes, and sponges clean because, when wet, they harbor bacteria and may promote bacterial growth. Wash dishcloths often in hot water in the washing machine and wash the sponges and brushes in the dishwasher once weekly.

- Sanitize the kitchen sink drain periodically by pouring a solution of 1 teaspoon of chlorine bleach to 1 quart of water or a commercial kitchen-cleaning agent down the drain. Food particles get trapped in the drain and garbage disposal and, along with the moisture, create an ideal environment for bacterial growth. *Campylobacter* has been found in kitchen drains.

- Use plastic cutting boards that are free of cracks and crevices. Avoid boards made of soft, porous materials such as wood. Wash cutting boards with hot water and soap, using a scrub brush. Then, sanitize them by washing in an automatic dishwasher or by rinsing with a solution of 1 teaspoon of chlorine bleach to 1 quart of water.

• Always wash and sanitize cutting boards after using them for raw foods, such as poultry or fish, and before using them for ready-to-eat foods. Consider using one cutting board only for foods that will be cooked, such as raw chicken, and another only for ready-to-eat foods, such as bread, fresh fruit, and cooked meats.

• Always use clean utensils and wash them between cutting different foods.

• Wash the lids of canned foods before opening to keep dirt from getting into the food. Also, clean the blade of the can opener after each use. Food processors and meat grinders should be taken apart and cleaned as soon as possible after they are used.

• Do not put cooked poultry on an unwashed plate or platter that has held raw poultry.

• Do not reuse marinades from raw poultry or meat.

Keep the Temperature Right

The second rule, after keeping everything clean, is to keep hot foods hot and cold foods cold.

• Use a food thermometer to ensure that meats are completely cooked. Insert the thermometer into the center of the food and wait 30 seconds to ensure an accurate measurement. (Quick-read thermometers require only a few seconds.) Beef, lamb, and veal should be cooked to at least 145°F (63°C); pork and ground beef to 160°F (71°C); whole poultry and thighs to 180°F (82°C); poultry breasts to 170°F (77°C); and ground chicken or turkey to 165°F (74°C). Thermometers with fast reading times and easy to read indicators (such as rare, medium rare, medium, well done, and poultry) are available today for less than $20. One of the easiest ways to avoid food poisoning, including campylobacteriosis, is to cook your food properly (Figure 7.2).

- If you do not have a food thermometer, buy one. Do not depend on how the food looks unless it is extremely well done (no pinkness in the juice at all).

- Poultry or meats can be cooked in the microwave. Just make sure the food reaches the correct temperature.

- Protect food from cross-contamination after cooking by keeping everything clean and eating it promptly.

- Cooked foods should not be left standing on the table or kitchen counter for more than two hours. Pathogenic bacteria grow in temperatures between 40° and 140°F (4° and 60°C) and remember that they grow exponentially, not linearly. *Campylobacter jejuni* thrives at 42°C (107.6°F). Cooked foods that have been in this temperature range for more than two hours should not be eaten.

- If food is to be served hot, get it from the stove to the table as quickly as possible. Reheated foods should be brought to a temperature of at least 165°F (74°C). Keep cold foods in the refrigerator or on a bed of ice until serving, particularly during the summer months.

- After the meal, leftovers should be refrigerated as soon as possible. Meats should be cut in slices of three inches or less and all foods should be stored in shallow containers to hasten cooling. Leftovers should be used within 3 to 4 days and reheated properly.

- Do not thaw poultry and other frozen foods at room temperature. Instead, move them from the freezer to the

FOOD	°F
Ground Meat & Meat Mixtures	
Beef, Pork, Veal, Lamb	160
Turkey, Chicken	165
Fresh Beef, Veal, Lamb	
Medium Rare	145
Medium	160
Well Done	170
Poultry	
Chicken & Turkey, whole	180
Poultry breasts, roast	170
Poultry thighs, wings	180
Duck & Goose	180
Stuffing (cooked alone or in bird)	165
Fresh Pork	
Medium	160
Well Done	170
Ham	
Fresh (raw)	160
Pre-cooked (to reheat)	140
Eggs & Egg Dishes	
Eggs	Cook until yolk & white are firm
Egg dishes	160
Leftovers & Casseroles	165

Figure 7.2 To kill harmful bacteria present in meat, poultry, and eggs, the food must be cooked to the proper temperature. The minimum safe cooking temperatures for common foods are listed in this chart.

refrigerator for 1 to 2 days or defrost submerged in cold water. You can also defrost in the microwave oven or during the cooking process. Cook foods immediately after defrosting in the microwave or cold water.

In Restaurants

- Be observant. If the restaurant is dirty, chances are that the kitchen is also dirty.

Additional Tips Pertaining to *Campylobacter*

- Do not drink untreated water, no matter how clean it looks.

- Do not drink unpasteurized milk.

- Since pets can spread *Campylobacter* to humans via their feces, wash your hands thoroughly with warm water and soap after contact with farm animals, dogs, cats, and their feces.

- Be extra cautious around animals with diarrhea, although animals can be healthy while providing a reservoir for *Campylobacter*.

Those who are more susceptible or immunocompromised must take the prevention tips seriously. This includes pregnant women, lactating women, infants, children, the elderly, and those whose immune systems are impaired. These include people undergoing chemo- or radiotherapy for cancer; those with heart disease, diabetes, liver or kidney disease, or AIDS; and those who are malnourished or under tremendous stress. When traveling, do not take chances. Drink treated water, ask where the water for the ice cubes came from, and do not eat anything raw.

These prevention tips may seem overwhelming at first, but with practice, they will become effortless habits. Prevention boils down to respecting temperature requirements and keeping everything clean. Purchase a thermometer, sanitize with bleach, wash your dishcloths often and toss your sponges and brushes in the dishwasher along with your dishes once a week.

In summary, although food has to go through many channels prior to reaching your table, as consumers, we can significantly impact the outcome by understanding the factors that influence bacterial growth and controlling those factors. Many infections have resulted from carelessness in our own kitchens. In this book about *Campylobacter* you have learned much about symptoms and complications to watch for, how campylobacteriosis spreads, how bacteria cause disease, and what you can do to prevent disease. These concepts apply to many microorganisms, including various bacteria, viruses, parasites, and fungi. Basic sanitary measures such as keeping everything clean and respecting temperature zones will serve you well in protecting you and your family from infectious diseases.

An absolutely risk-free food supply does not exist. As consumers, we must accept some responsibility for keeping our food safe.

Glossary

Aerobic bacteria—Bacteria that require oxygen for their metabolism.

Amoebas—Any of the protozoa under the Order Amoebida.

Anaerobes—Bacteria that do not require oxygen for their metabolism.

Anaerobic—Living or existing in the absence of oxygen.

Antibiotic—A compound that is capable of inhibiting or killing microorganisms.

Antibody—A protein produced by the immune system in response to an antigen.

Antigen—A foreign substance or microorganism that elicits an immune response when introduced into the body.

Appendicitis—Inflammation of the appendix.

Arthropod—Any member of the Phylum Arthropoda, which includes all members with a skeletal covering composed of chitin.

Asymptomatic—Not displaying any disease symptoms.

Avirulent—Not virulent.

Bacteremia—The condition that results when bacteria are present in the bloodstream.

Bacteremic shock—Shock caused by high levels of bacteria in the bloodstream.

Bacteriological incubator—Specific incubator with a controlled environment produced to promote the growth of bacteria.

Bacteriophage—Virus that infects bacteria.

Bacterium—A unicellular, prokaryotic organism of the Kingdom Monera.

B cell—Lymphocyte cell that produces antibodies.

Bile salts—Greenish-yellowish secretion produced by the liver, stored, and secreted by the gallbladder into the small intestine to help digest fats.

Blood pressure—The force exerted by the blood on the walls of the blood vessels, measured in systolic (highest) over diastolic (lowest) force; normal blood pressure is around 120/80.

Bowel movement—The act of eliminating feces and other waste materials.

Campylobacteriosis—The infectious disease caused by the bacterium *Campylobacter*.

Capsid—The protein coat covering viruses.

Cell division—The process by which a mother cell divides into two identical daughter cells.

Cellular—Referring to the cellular level (e.g., changes to the cell).

Chromosome—Thread-like structure containing the genetic material (DNA or RNA).

Cilia—Hair-like structures forming part of a fringe on the surface of a microorganism, which allow unicellular organisms such as bacteria or protozoa to move. In eukaryotes, cilia allow movement of mucus, as in the respiratory tract.

Ciliate—Any ciliated protozoa.

Clinical diagnosis—A diagnosis made strictly on the basis of the knowledge of the physician, obtained via medical history and physical examination without the help of laboratory tests or X-rays.

Clinical symptoms—Changes in the body's condition as perceived by the patient.

Coccoid bodies—The shape that bacteria take when, under stressful conditions, certain bacteria curl up and appear round under a microscope.

Colitis—Inflammation of the colon; if severe, lesions or ulcers are present.

Colonization—Condition when bacteria multiply and flourish at a particular site.

Colony—Mass of cells derived from a single cell.

Commensals—Organisms that derive benefits from another organism without causing harm to the host organism.

Competitive exclusion—When different species compete for the same place in the ecosystem, and one thrives, leaving the other to die or find another ecological niche.

Complement system—A group of proteins that mediate the inflammatory system and are involved in opsonization.

Congenital malformation—Any abnormality of an infant present at the time of birth.

Glossary

Conjugation—A form of DNA transfer that involves direct cell-to-cell contact via a sex pilus.

Cross-contamination—The transfer of microorganisms from something that is contaminated to something that is not.

Cyst—In humans, a cyst is an enclosed sac within body tissues with a distinct membrane. In parasitic worms, cysts develop around the larval form within the tissue of the host animal. In adverse conditions, protozoa form cysts by secreting a wall around themselves and living in a hibernated state.

Cytoplasm—The substance outside of the nucleus of eukaryotes and the substance filling the cells of prokaryotes.

Definitive diagnosis—A diagnosis that has been confirmed by laboratory tests or X-rays.

Deoxyribonucleic acid (DNA)—Contains the genetic information required for the transmission of inherited traits.

Diagnosis—See **Clinical diagnosis**.

Disease—Existence of pathology, which is any abnormality caused by an infection.

Disinfectant—Any substance applied to inanimate objects to kill microorganisms.

Duodenum—The first part of the small intestine; receives food from the stomach and begins the absorption of nutrients.

Endotoxin—A toxic component of the Gram-negative membrane that is released when the bacterium ruptures or dies.

Enteritis—Inflammation of the intestines; if severe, lesions or ulcers result.

Enzyme—A substance that catalyzes (brings about or incites) a reaction without being altered in the process.

Eukaryotic—Any organism that possesses cells with a clearly defined nucleus composed of a nuclear membrane, which encloses the chromosomes (DNA or RNA).

Excystment—The process of forming a cyst.

Fecal-oral route—Route of transmission from ingestion of foods contaminated by feces.

Flagella—Whip-like structures attached to a basal body in the cell wall that allows locomotion.

Flora—Microorganisms that are naturally found in certain areas of the body.

Foodborne illness—Disease caused by ingestion of contaminated foods.

Fungi—Any of the organisms in the Kingdom Fungi, including mushrooms, yeasts, molds, and mildews.

Gastroenteritis—A syndrome in which the lining of the stomach and intestine become inflamed, causing abdominal cramps and diarrhea.

Golgi apparatus—Structure in a cell that is responsible for modifying, completing, and exporting proteins.

Gram stain—Microbiological staining technique that helps characterize bacteria based on the differentiation of cell walls.

Helminthes—Parasitic worms.

Hemoglobin—Protein in red blood cells that transports oxygen to the tissues. When oxygenated, hemoglobin is bright red; when not oxygenated, it is purplish blue.

Hemorrhage—A loss of a large amount of blood in a short period of time.

Immunocompromised—People whose immune systems are impaired or weakened, due either to disease or an inherited condition.

Immunodeficient—See **Immunocompromised**.

Incidence—Rate of occurrence.

Incubation period—The time between exposure of a pathogen and the onset of symptoms of a disease.

Infection—The invasion of the body by a pathogen that multiplies and causes disease.

Infectious disease—Any disease that can be transmitted from one human being to another or from an animal to a human.

Infective dose—The dose required for infection to occur.

Inflammation—A defense response by the immune system triggered by damage to living tissues.

Intermediate host—Host that transfers a parasite from one host to another, but is not the final host.

Glossary

Intoxication—The condition that occurs when pathogens produce a toxin in the food that causes the disease.

Larvae—Stage in the development of organisms, occurring after birth and prior to the adult form; an immature form.

Life cycle—Series of changes that organisms undergo as they pass through various developmental stages.

Lipopolysaccharide (LPS)—See **Endotoxin**.

Lymphocytes—White blood cells that are involved in the immune response, including B cells and T cells.

Lymphoid system—Also called the lymphatic system. A subsystem of the circulatory system that is responsible for fluid balance and drainage and for producing and maturing lymphocytes.

Lysosomes—Organelles inside eukaryotic cells responsible for the cell's digestion of macromolecules, microorganisms, and old cell parts; has an acidic environment surrounded by its own membrane.

Macrophage—A type of white blood cell or leukocyte, the mature form of a monocyte that both lives free and resides in tissues and is capable of phagocytosis and cell signaling.

Media—Solution containing the substances required for the growth of microorganisms that can be liquid or solidified with agar.

Microaerophilic—Microorganisms that grow better in low concentrations of oxygen.

Mitochondria—Organelles inside the cell that are responsible for the production of energy (often called the powerhouses of the cell).

Molecular microbiology—Study of the structures and processes of microbiological activities at the molecular level, including the study of proteins, nucleic acids such as DNA, and enzymes, and how these molecules function and interact.

Nomenclature—A system of naming organisms based on concise and accurate descriptions so that scientists internationally can recognize and agree to a standard name for an organism; refers to the genus and species of an organism.

Nonspecific defense system—Host defenses (which include physical barriers, phagocytic cells, complement, and inflammatory response) that are always present and repel all pathogens equally; are effective against most pathogens.

Nucleus—Carries the genes (DNA in chromosomes) in eukaryotic cells and is enveloped by a double layer called the nuclear membrane.

Opportunistic pathogen—A pathogen that does not affect healthy people but affects those who are immunocompromised.

Opsonization—Process by which complement proteins bind to invading organisms, marking them for ingestion by phagocytes.

Oral rehydration therapy—An oral fluid replacement recipe used by world aid workers to increase the body's ability to absorb fluid by 25-fold. A common recipe is 1 cup treated water, 2 teaspoons sugar, and a pinch of salt.

Parasite—Organism that thrives at the expense of another organism (the host) without killing it; can cause significant abnormalities in the host organism.

Pasteurization—Treatment of milk or juice with sufficient heat to kill certain disease-causing microorganisms and to decrease the levels of bacteria to an acceptable level; not a sterilization process.

Pathogen—Microorganism capable of causing disease.

Pathology—Medical field concerned with determining the cause of disease.

Peptidoglycan—Structure in cell walls that gives bacteria their shape.

Perinatal infection—Infection occurring during pregnancy or at the time of birth.

Peristalsis—Wavelike muscular movements in the digestive tract that move the intestinal contents through the digestive tract.

pH—A measure of acidity. A pH of 7 is neutral, a pH of 1 is strongly acidic, and a pH of 14 is strongly basic (alkaline).

Phagocytes—White blood cells of the immune system whose function is to engulf and destroy pathogens.

Phagocytosis—Process of phagocytes engulfing invaders.

Photosynthesis—Process by which plants convert light energy to chemical energy.

Glossary

Placenta—Organ in which fetal and maternal blood circulates in close proximity in the uterus in order to exchange nutrients, oxygen, and wastes.

Placental insufficiency—A condition that occurs when there is insufficient transfer of oxygen, nutrients, or wastes between the mother and fetus.

Prodrome—A premonitory symptom that warns of impending disease.

Prokaryote—Unicellular organism lacking a distinct nucleus. Chromosomes are dispersed in cytoplasm; organelles such as Golgi bodies and lysosomes are not present.

Protozoa—Any member of the subkingdom Protozoa consisting of unicellular eukaryotic organisms.

Pseudopodia—Extensions of the cytoplasm of the organism, allowing amoeboid movement.

Pulse—The regular expansion and contraction of an artery caused by waves of pressure from the contraction of the heart. An average pulse for an adult is 60–80 beats per minute.

Receptors—Cells or groups of cells whose function is to bind to specific molecules to elicit a response.

Relapse—A recurrence of symptoms.

Reservoir—An organism in which a parasite that is pathogenic for another species inhabits and reproduces without damaging the host.

Sanitize—To decrease the number of microorganisms to a safe level. Chlorine bleach is commonly used to sanitize countertops and machinery.

Septicemia—Disease where microorganisms are multiplying in the blood and toxins are being released by the bacteria.

Sex pilus—Projection allowing one bacterium to adhere to another in a mating process called conjugation, in which DNA is transferred from one bacterium to the other.

Shock—A shut-down of the body systems, which occurs when the circulatory system fails to supply enough blood to peripheral tissues, resulting in inadequate oxygenation and removal of wastes.

Side effect—Consequence resulting from medication or therapy that is usually undesirable, such as constipation, dry mouth, or dizziness.

Specific defense system—Host defenses produced in response to an invasion by a specific pathogen; includes B cells, T cells, and antibodies.

Spore—A resistant form of bacteria produced during adverse conditions.

Stool sample—A sample of the feces of a patient to be sent to the laboratory for testing.

Susceptible populations—Subpopulations of humans that are more susceptible to disease, including infants and children, pregnant and lactating women, the elderly, and the immunocompromised.

Symptoms—See **Clinical symptoms**.

T cells—Lymphocyte cells that kill host cells that have been infected by pathogens, activate macrophages, and stimulate B cells to produce antibodies.

Transduction—A form of DNA transfer that occurs when a type of virus (a bacteriophage) attacks a bacterium.

Transformation—A form of DNA transfer that occurs when cells take up the DNA in the environment from dead cells.

Ulcerative colitis—A chronic disease characterized by severe inflammation of the colon and rectum with ulcers in the inflamed membrane.

Ulcers—Lesions in an inflamed area resulting from necrosis (tissue death); can be shallow or deep.

Vascular—Containing a blood supply.

Vectors—Transmitter of pathogens.

Virulence—Ability of an organism to cause disease.

Viruses—Any member of the Kingdom Virus; organisms that cannot reproduce without the aid of other cells.

White blood cell—Cellular component of the blood that lacks hemoglobin and defends the body against infection.

Zoonosis—Any disease shared by humans and other vertebrate animals (animals with backbones).

Zoonotic disease—Refers to a disease that can be transmitted from animals to humans.

Notes

1. Sizer, F., and E. Whitney. *Nutrition, Concepts and Controversies,* 8th Ed. Belmont, CA: Wadsworth, Thomson Learning, 2000.

2. Food Safety and Inspection Service, United States Department of Agriculture. "Campylobacter questions and Answers." Available online at *http://www.fsis.usda. gov/OA/background/campyq&a.htm.*

3. Deming, M.S., R.V. Tauxe, P.A. Blake, S.E. Dixon, B.S. Fowler, T.S. Jones, E.A. Lockamy, C.M. Patton, and R.O. Sikes. "*Campylobacter* enteritis at a university: transmission from eating chicken and from cats." *American Journal of Epidemiology.* 126(1987): 526–534.

4. Harrington, P., J. Archer, J.P. Davis, D.R. Croft, and J.K. Varma. "Outbreak of *Campylobacter jejuni* Infections Associated with Drinking Unpasteurized Milk Procured through a Cow-Leasing Program—Wisconsin, 2001." *MMWR Weekly.* 51 (June 28, 2002): 548–549. Available online at *http://www.cdc.gov/ mmwr/preview/mmwrhtml/mm5125a2. htm.*

5. Nachamkin, I., and M.J. Blaser, eds. *Campylobacter,* 2nd Ed. Washington, D.C.: ASM Press, 2000.

6. Ibid.

7. Ibid.

8. Sizer and Whitney, 2000.

9. Nachamkin and Blaser, 2000.

10. Ibid.

11. Konkel, M.E., S.G. Garvis, S.L. Tipton, D.E. Anderson, Jr., and W. Cieplak, Jr. "Identification and molecular cloning of a gene encoding a fibronectin-binding protein (CadF) from *Campylobacter jejuni.*" *Molecular Microbiology.* 24 (1997): 953–963.

12. Bereswill, S., and M. Kist. "Molecular microbiology and pathogenesis of *Helicobacter* and *Campylobacter* updated: a meeting report of the 11th conference on *Campylobacter, Helicobacter* and related organisms." *Molecular Microbiology.* 45 (2002): 255–262.

13. Konkel, M.E., B.J. Kim, V. Rivera-Amill, and S.G. Garvis. "Bacterial secreted proteins are required for the internalization of *Campylobacter jejuni* into cultured mammalian cells." *Molecular Microbiology.* 32(1999): 691–701.

14. Day, W.A., J.L. Sajecki, T.M. Pitts, and L.A. Joens. "Role of Catalase in *Campylobacter jejuni* Intracellular Survival." *Infection and Immunity.* 68(2000): 6337–6345.

15. Ibid.

16. Mead, P.S., L. Slutsker, V. Dietz, L.F. McCaig, J.S. Bresee, C. Shapiro, P.M. Griffin, and R. Tauxe. "Food-Related Illness and Death in the United States." *Emerging Infectious Diseases* [serial online] September–October 5, 1999 (5). Available online at *http://www.cdc.gov/ ncidod/eid/vol5no5/mead.htm.*

Bibliography

Altman, L.J. *Plague and Pestilence: A History of Infectious Disease.* Berkeley Heights, NJ: Enslow Publishers, Inc., 1998.

Baron, Samuel, ed. *Medical Microbiology,* 4th Ed. Galveston, TX: The University of Texas Medical Branch at Galveston, 1996.

Bereswill, S., and M. Kist. "Molecular microbiology and pathogenesis of *Helicobacter* and *Campylobacter* updated: a meeting report of the 11th conference on *Campylobacter, Helicobacter* and related organisms." *Molecular Microbiology.* 45 (2002): 255–262.

Bogitsh, B.J., and T.C. Cheng. *Human Parasitology,* 2nd Ed. San Diego, CA: Academic Press, 1998.

Day, Nancy. *Killer Superbugs: The Story of Drug-Resistant Diseases.* Berkeley Heights, NJ: Enslow Publishers, Inc., 2001.

Day, W.A., J.L. Sajecki, T.M. Pitts, and L.A. Joens. "Role of Catalase in *Campylobacter jejuni* Intracellular Survival." *Infection and Immunity* 68 (2000): 6337–6345.

Deming, M.S., R.V. Tauxe, P.A. Blake, S.E. Dixon, B.S. Fowler, T.S. Jones, E.A. Lockamy, C.M. Patton, and R.O. Sikes. "*Campylobacter* enteritis at a university: transmission from eating chicken and from cats." *American Journal of Epidemiology* 126(1987): 526–534.

Egendorf, L.K. *Food Safety.* Farmington Hills, MI: Gale Group, 1999.

Ewald, P.M. *Evolution of Infectious Disease.* New York: Oxford University Press, 1996.

Flint, S.J., L.W. Enquist, R.M. Krug, V.R. Racaniello, and A.M. Skalka. *Principles of Virology: Molecular Biology, Pathogenesis, and Control.* Washington, D.C.: ASM Press, 1999.

Forrest, K.V., J.H. Jorgensen, and P.R. Murray. *Manual of Clinical Microbiology,* 8th Ed. Washington, D.C.: ASM Press, 2003.

Garrett, Laurie. *The Coming Plague: Newly Emerging Diseases in a World Out of Balance.* New York: Penguin USA, 1995.

Harrington, P., J. Archer, J.P. Davis, D.R. Croft, and J.K. Varma. "Outbreak of *Campylobacter jejuni* Infections Associated with Drinking Unpasteurized Milk Procured through a Cow-Leasing Program—Wisconsin, 2001." *MMWR Weekly* 51 (June 28, 2002): 548–549. Available online at *http://www.cdc.gov/mmwr/preview/mmwrhtml/mm5125a2.htm.*

Bibliography

Konkel, M.E., B.J. Kim, V. Rivera-Amill, and S.G. Garvis. "Bacterial secreted proteins are required for the internalization of *Campylobacter jejuni* into cultured mammalian cells." *Molecular Microbiology* 32(1999): 691–701.

Konkel, M.E., S.G. Garvis, S.L. Tipton, D.E. Anderson, Jr., and W. Cieplak, Jr. "Identification and molecular cloning of a gene encoding a fibronectin-binding protein (CadF) from *Campylobacter jejuni*." *Molecular Microbiology* 24 (1997): 953–963.

Maier, Raina M., Ian L. Pepper, and Charles P. Gerba. *Environmental Microbiology*. San Diego: Academic Press, 2000.

Mead, P.S., L. Slutsker, V. Dietz, L.F. McCaig, J.S. Bresee, C. Shapiro, P.M. Griffin, and R. Tauxe. "Food-Related Illness and Death in the United States." *Emerging Infectious Diseases* [serial online] September–October 5, 1999 (5). Available online at *http://www.cdc.gov/ncidod/eid/vol5no5/mead.htm*.

Nachamkin, I., and M.J. Blaser, eds. *Campylobacter*, 2nd Ed. Washington, D.C.: ASM Press, 2000.

Nourse, A.E., and V. Mathews, eds. *Virus Invaders*. Danbury, CT: Franklin Watts, 1992.

Roitt, Ivan M., Jonathan Brostoff, and David Male, eds. *Immunology*, 6th Ed. St. Louis, MO: Mosby, Inc., 2001.

Salyers, Abigail A., and Dixie D. Whitt. *Bacterial Pathogenesis—A Molecular Approach*, 2nd Ed. Washington, D.C.: ASM Press, 2002.

Sizer, F., and E. Whitney. *Nutrition, Concepts and Controversies*, 8th Ed. Belmont, CA: Wadsworth, Thomson Learning, 2000.

Websites

For excellent information on any diseases or bacteria,
go to the homepage of CDC and type in a search.

Federal Organizations Involved in Food Protection and Public Safety

Centers for Disease Control and Prevention (CDC)
http://www.cdc.gov

Food and Drug Administration (FDA)
http://www.fda.gov

FDA's Center for Food Safety and Applied Nutrition (CFSAN)
http://www.cfsan.fda.gov/list.html

United States Department of Agriculture (USDA)
http://www.usda.gov

General Disease Information

Bacterial and Fungal Diseases (CDC)
http://www.cdc.gov/ncidod/dbmd/diseaseinfo/default.htm

Food Safety and Inspection Service,
Campylobacter Questions and Answers
http://www.fsis.usda.gov/OA/background/campyq&a.htm

Parasites and Parasitic Diseases (CDC)
http://www.dpd.cdc.gov

Viral Diseases (CDC)
http://www.cdc.gov/ncidod/dvrd/index.htm

Bacteria

Bad Bug Book (CFSAN)
http://www.cfsan.fda.gov/~mow/intro.html

Microbiology
http://www.microbeworld.org/home.htm

Sizes of cells, bacteria, viruses
http://www.cellsalive.com/howbig.htm

Websites

Prevention

Consumer Advice from FDA's Center for
Food Safety and Applied Nutrition (CFSAN)
http://vm.cfsan.fda.gov/~lrd/advice.html

FDA's Unwelcome Dinner Guest Website
http://www.cfsan.fda.gov/~dms/fdunwelc.html

Food Safety
http://www.foodsafety.gov

USDA's Home Canning Information
http://www.agen.ufl.edu/~foodsaf/can1.html

Statistics

CDC's Mortality and Morbidity Weekly Reports (MMWR)
http://www.cdc.gov/mmwr/about.html

Foodnet
http://www.cdc.gov/foodnet/default.htm

Index

Index

Picture Credits

15: Information from *Morbidity and Mortality Weekly Report*, Vol 52, no. 15, CDC

18: Lambda Science Artwork

22: Lambda Science Artwork

25: Lambda Science Artwork

26: © Gladden Willis/Visuals Unlimited

28: (top) Courtesy Public Health Image Library (PHIL), CDC

28: (bottom) © Michael Abbey/ Visuals Unlimited

36: © Dr. Gary Gaugler/Visuals Unlimited

39: © Carolina Biological/Visuals Unlimited

53: Lambda Science Artwork

57: © Larry Stepanowicz/Visuals Unlimited

62: © Dr. Veronika Burmeister/ Visuals Unlimited

63: Lambda Science Artwork

67: © Dr. Donald Fawcett & E. Shelton/ Visuals Unlimited

71: Photo by Anna Bates, Courtesy Agricultural Research Service, USDA

80: (top) Courtesy USDA

80: (bottom) © Bernard Wittich/ Visuals Unlimited

85: Courtesy USDA

91: Information from USDA

Cover: © Dr. Gary Gaugler/Visuals Unlimited

About the Author

Bibiana Law is presently studying at the University of Arizona for her doctoral degree on the virulence traits and pathogenicity of *Campylobacter jejuni* in chickens. The project is funded by USDA and the university. She is a graduate research associate in the Department of Soil, Water and Environmental Sciences. Furthermore, she is an instructor for the Department of Nutritional Sciences. She holds a Bachelor's degree in Nutritional Sciences from McGill University in Montreal, Canada, from which she graduated as the top student in the department. Bibiana has been honored with more than a dozen awards including medals, scholarships, and prizes for her outstanding academic achievement. She is happily married to her loving husband and resides in Tucson, Arizona.

About the Editor

The late I. Edward Alcamo was a Distinguished Teaching Professor of Microbiology at the State University of New York at Farmingdale. Alcamo studied biology at Iona College in New York and earned his M.S. and Ph.D. degrees in microbiology at St. John's University, also in New York. He had taught at Farmingdale for over 30 years. In 2000, Alcamo won the Carski Award for Distinguished Teaching in Microbiology, the highest honor for microbiology teachers in the United States. He was a member of the American Society for Microbiology, the National Association of Biology Teachers, and the American Medical Writers Association. Alcamo authored numerous books on the subjects of microbiology, AIDS, and DNA technology as well as the award-winning textbook *Fundamentals of Microbiology*, now in its sixth edition.